WHY YOU SHOULD READ THIS BOOK

Like most of us today, you probably have to carve out time in your busy schedule in order to read a book. Therefore, you don't want your time to be wasted, and you want what you read to have value for you. If you are thinking of reading this book, you are most likely interested in finding answers for how you can improve your health and the health of your loved ones. I wrote this book to help you do so.

Over the course of many years, as both a writer of health books and an explorer of effective self-care measures that we can all use to improve our health, I have discovered that many of the most effective solutions are to be found in nature. Such natural solutions not only offer important health benefits but are also inexpensive and readily available—and can be as effective as any prescription or over-the-counter medication. And, as an added advantage, they are also free of the unpleasant, even dangerous, side effects so commonly caused by pharmaceutical drugs today. As this book makes clear, that is certainly the case for turmeric and its primary ingredient, curcumin.

If you read this book to its end and, most importantly, if you apply the suggestions for improving your health that it offers on a consistent basis, I promise you that your time will not be wasted and that there is a very good chance you will find beneficial answers to your health concerns that will make a positive difference in your life.

Thank you for choosing to read it.

OTHER WORKS BY LARRY TRIVIERI, JR.

From Square One Publishers

Coconuts for Your Health

Apple Cider Vinegar: Nature's Most Powerful and Versatile Remedy

*The Acid-Alkaline Lifestyle: The Complete Program
for Better Health and Vitality* (with Neil Raff, MD)

The Acid-Alkaline Food Guide (with Susan Brown, PhD)

Juice Alive: The Ultimate Guide to Juicing Remedies
(with Steven Bailey, ND)

Other Select Titles

The American Medical Association Guide to Holistic Health

Alternative Medicine: The Definitive Guide, 1st and 2nd editions
(editor and co-author with Burton Goldberg)

Chronic Fatigue, Fibromyalgia and Lyme Disease
(with Burton Goldberg)

Novels

The Monster and Freddie Fype

Krystle's Quest

Tommy's Big Question

TURMERIC
FOR YOUR HEALTH

*Nature's Most Powerful
Anti-Inflammatory*

Larry Trivieri, Jr.

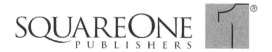

SQUAREONE
PUBLISHERS

The information and advice contained in this book are based upon the research and the personal and professional experiences of the authors. They are not intended as a substitute for consulting with a health care professional. The publisher and author are not responsible for any adverse effects or consequences resulting from the use of any of the suggestions, preparations, or procedures discussed in this book. All matters pertaining to your physical health should be supervised by a health care professional. It is a sign of wisdom, not cowardice, to seek a second or third opinion.

EDITOR: Erica Shur
COVER DESIGNER: Jeannie Tudor
TYPESETTER: Gary A. Rosenberg

Square One Publishers
115 Herricks Road
Garden City Park, NY 11040
(516) 535-2010 • (877) 900-BOOK
www.squareonepublishers.com

Library of Congress Cataloging-in-Publication Data

Names: Larry Trivieri, Jr., author.
Title: Turmeric for your health / Larry Trivieri, Jr.
Description: Garden City Park, NY : Square One Publishers, [2018] | Includes bibliographical references.
Identifiers: LCCN 2018008328 | ISBN 0757004520 (pbk.)
Subjects: LCSH: Turmeric—Therapeutic use. | Turmeric—Health aspects.
Classification: LCC RS165.T8 L37 2018 | DDC 615.3/2488—dc23
LC record available at https://lccn.loc.gov/2018008328

Printed in the United States of America

10   9   8   7   6   5   4   3   2   1

Contents

This one is for Bryan Herman,
my nephew, my friend, and all-around class act.

Introduction

Cancer.

Heart disease.

Alzheimer's disease and dementia.

Diabetes.

Arthritis and joint pain.

Gastrointestinal diseases.

As we progress through the twenty-first century, the above conditions are among the most common scourges affecting our lives today. Combined, they account for much of the over three trillion dollars that the United States spends each year on health care. But the full toll of such conditions far exceeds their financial costs alone. More importantly, they rob those who suffer from them, as well as their loved ones, of a long, healthy, high-quality life. And compounding the problem is the fact that our modern health care system is no closer to providing real solutions for dealing with these conditions. For the most part, all that it offers are drugs to manage the symptoms of these diseases and little more. Not only do such drugs often fail to provide complete relief, they can also be costly and result in a wide array of potential side effects. Clearly, we are in need of better solutions for these problems.

In recognition of this fact, a growing number of physicians and researchers alike are turning away from drug-based symptom care and are rediscovering what ancient healers across the globe taught. Namely, that our health depends first and foremost on the foods we eat, and that nature has provided us with an abundance of herbs and spices that not only enhance the flavors of these foods, but also provide significant health benefits.

In this book, I am going to share with you information about one of the most powerful of these herbs and spices: turmeric. In the pages that follow, you will learn how and why turmeric and its primary ingredient, curcumin, can make a big difference in your overall health and help reduce the risk of the diseases previously mentioned above, as well as other health conditions. Specifically, you will learn:

- What turmeric is, and why for millennia it has been recommended as a medicinal spice by the healing traditions of both China and India.

- How turmeric and curcumin act to protect against chronic inflammation, a primary cause of up to 90 percent of all health conditions today.

- The exciting possibilities turmeric holds for preventing Alzheimer's disease and dementia.

- Why researchers are so excited about turmeric's potential as a cancer-fighter.

- How turmeric can protect against heart disease.

- Why turmeric can be helpful for people with diabetes.

- The reasons why turmeric can help prevent and soothe symptoms of arthritis and joint pain.

- What you need to know to get the most benefit from turmeric and turmeric supplements.

So, if you are ready to add more spice to your health, keep reading.

1

The Healing Spice

For centuries, turmeric has been regarded as a healing spice by people in China, India, and other Asian countries. This is because the two major healing traditions of those countries—Ayurvedic medicine (also known as Ayurveda) and traditional Chinese medicine (TCM)—recognized turmeric's medicinal properties long before the advent of the medical traditions here in the West. As a result, in these Asian countries, turmeric is a common ingredient in many food dishes, such as curry. It is also used in tea and other tonic drinks.

Both Ayurveda and TCM originated at least 3,000 years ago, in India and China, respectively. What is so fascinating to me about both healing systems is how comprehensive they are in scope. Dating back to their early origins, both systems recognized the need to address both health and disease from the perspective of what holistic physicians today term "body, mind, and spirit." As a result, in both traditions one can find equal emphasis given to diet, nutrition, physical exercise, and the care of the emotions, as well as meditation and other contemplative practices.

Just as important, both Ayurveda and TCM recognize the existence of a vitalizing life force energy. In Ayurveda, this life force is known as *prana*. In TCM, it is called *Qi* (pronounced "chee"). Both traditions also recognize the existence of unseen energy pathways in the body (known as meridians in TCM, and *nadis* and *chakras* in Ayurveda), and how energetic imbalances or blockages within these pathways are a primary cause of disease.

Additionally, both traditions realized from their onset that a "one size fits all" approach to healing, which is still a hallmark of modern medicine in the West to a large extent, is inappropriate given the unique needs of each person. In recognition of this fact, Ayurvedic physicians treat patients according to their *dosha,* or what today in the West is known as their "specific metabolic type." TCM practitioners treat their patients according to the balance or imbalance of five elements (wood, fire, earth, metal, and water) within each person, as well as whether they have an excess or deficiency of *yin* or *yang*, the feminine and masculine components of *Qi*. Until the late twentieth century, however, Western conventional medicine and science rejected both systems of medicine as being largely based on unproven superstitions. Fortunately, that has begun to change.

The impetus for that change largely began in the 1970s. At that time, studies conducted at the famed Menninger Clinic and other research institutions demonstrated the powerful benefits that components of Ayurvedic medicine, such as meditation and yoga, have for improving health and preventing and reversing disease. During that same time, Western physicians and researchers began to take an interest in acupuncture and other aspects of TCM.

Since that time, Western scientists have gone on to confirm the existence of the human body's energy field and energetic pathways, while an increasing number of physicians have turned to diet and nutrition as primary tools for helping to keep their patients healthy. In addition, just as Ayurvedic and TCM physicians have done for centuries, Western doctors have learned how to tailor diets to each patient's specific metabolic type. In place of the diagnostic methods developed under Ayurveda and TCM, today's physicians do so through the use of various tests and genetic markers, but the results are often uncannily similar to what practitioners of these two ancient healing systems also achieve. Modern science is now, too, continuing to validate the health benefits of many other aspects of both Ayurveda and TCM, including the medicinal properties of the healing herbs and spices that, for centuries, have been part of the repertoire of both systems of healing.

This is especially true of turmeric, as evidenced by the vast number of scientific studies that have now been published in medical journals about its healing properties. In preparing my research for this book, I entered the term "turmeric" in Google Scholar. Over 98,000 entries came up, attesting to how widely and extensively it has been studied. Clearly then, turmeric is a natural healing agent that it is worth knowing about. So let's take a closer look at what turmeric is, its history of use, and why it can be so beneficial to your health.

WHAT IS TURMERIC?

Though you may be familiar with turmeric as a spice in curry dishes, if you are like me before I began to investigate it, you may not know much about it beyond its pleasant taste and bright yellow-orange appearance. Chances are you are far more familiar with ginger root, the plant to which it is closely related.

Like ginger, turmeric belongs to the plant family known as *Zingiberaceae*. Both turmeric and ginger are tropical perennial plants whose beneficial components are primarily found in their *rhizomes*, or roots. While both plants are highly regarded as healing spices in both Ayurveda and TCM, they have different properties, and are also different in terms of their taste and color once they are cut open (on the outside, ginger and turmeric are similar in appearance).

In the science of botany, turmeric is known as *Curcuma longa*, the name and classification given to it by the eighteenth-century botanist, zoologist, and physician Carl Linnaeus (1701–1778), who is credited with developing the modern-day system of classifying plants and other living organisms (taxonomy). In appearance, turmeric has a short stem and large, elongated leaves, with roots that are often multi-branched and brownish-yellow. When fully grown, the average turmeric plant is slightly more than three feet in height. Once harvested, its rhizome is dried and powdered to produce turmeric spice, which is used as a main ingredient in both curry and mustard.

The turmeric plant is native to both China and India, as well as other South Asian countries. Today, it is also grown and harvested in the Caribbean and parts of Latin America. In addition to its centuries-long use as a spice and medicinal herb in the Asian countries to which it is indigenous, turmeric is also used as a food coloring and preservative, and as a dye. Farmers in the region use it as a natural pesticide to protect their crops. In India, it is incorporated into religious (Hindu) ceremonies. Medicinally, turmeric has long been utilized as a powder, tincture, or tea, and also as a paste to treat such conditions as chicken pox, small pox, and measles.

As I mentioned above, in both Ayurveda and TCM, turmeric is recommended as a treatment for a wide range of disease conditions, and has been for thousands of years. Such diseases include digestive and gastrointestinal disorders, inflammatory diseases, respiratory problems, and conditions affecting the liver and gallbladder, including gallstones and other bile duct stones, cirrhosis, and jaundice. It has also been used traditionally to treat wounds, including wounds related to diabetes, and as an aid for injuries such as bruising, muscle pain, and sprains. As you will discover in reading through the rest of this book, modern science is now confirming turmeric's usefulness in helping to treat such conditions, as well as modern-day scourges such as cancer and Alzheimer's disease.

One other interesting fact about turmeric is that it is safe to consume at fairly high doses without posing any threat of toxicity. In India, the average daily consumption of turmeric is between 2 to 2.5 grams because of how commonly it is used as a spice in traditional Indian dishes, but it can safely be consumed at higher doses—although in some cases, such doses may result in gastrointestinal discomfort.

Turmeric: A Brief History

Turmeric was first cultivated nearly five thousand years ago in India, where it was used medicinally, and as both a spice and flavoring agent. It was also used as an offering to Hindu deities and applied to the foreheads of worshippers as a sign of purification. During that same time period, turmeric was written about in the early texts of Ayurvedic medicine, and is still used today by Ayurvedic physicians as an aid for preventing and reversing a variety of health conditions. According to Ayruvedic texts, there are more than 100 terms for turmeric that attest to its healing properties. For example, it is sometimes referred to a *jayanti,* which is also another name for the Hindu goddess Durga. Jayanti means "she who is victorious." In the case of turmeric, jayanti means "victorious over disease."

In the Hindu religion, turmeric is considered to be an auspicious and sacred spice and is used in various religious ceremonies. During the traditional Hindu wedding ceremony, for example, the groom will often tie a string has been dyed with turmeric around his bride's neck to signify that the bride is now married and worthy of overseeing the couple's household. According to Hindu tradition, wearing a piece of turmeric root as an amulet can also protect against evil spirits. In some parts of India, children often wear turmeric-dyed robes during celebrations of the Hindu god Krishna.

Because of its high regard in Indian culture, it is not surprising that India grows and harvests more of the turmeric plant each year than any other country, accounting for approximately 80 percent of the world's annual turmeric production, and about 60 percent of all turmeric exports.

With the dawn of Buddhism in India more than 2,500 years ago, turmeric began to be used as a dye to give the robes of Buddhist monks their characteristic yellowish-orange color. It is possible that it was the spread of Buddhism into China and other parts of Asia that brought turmeric and its various uses to the attention of the peoples in those countries. In any event, before long, turmeric was also being used as a healing spice by practitioners of traditional Chinese medicine.

In the West, turmeric was largely unknown until many centuries later. One of the first written records mentioning it came from Marco Polo (1254–1324), in his account of his travels through China and other parts of Asia. He wrote that turmeric had all the qualities of saffron, a spice that was highly prized at the time, with the only difference being that turmeric spice comes from the root of the turmeric plant, whereas saffron is derived from a flower (*Crocus sativus*).

For the most part, however, turmeric was largely ignored in the West, given that it is not indigenous to this part of the world. By the eighteenth century, though, its use as a spice in Western cooking began to appear, as evidenced by such cookbooks as *The Art of Cookery Made Plain and Easy*. This book was published in 1747 by Hannah Glasse (1708–1770), a popular English culinary author. It was so popular that it went through twenty editions and was still being published well into the nineteenth century. In the book, Glasse wrote of using turmeric to make a pickled Indian dish, and also included it in her recipe for curry. Around this same time, immigrants from India and other parts of Asia, where turmeric had long been used, began to arrive in England, bringing the spice with them. It is likely that Glasse became aware of turmeric and Indian cuisine because of this.

During the 1700s, a number of English merchants also began selling and advertising turmeric spice. Evidence of this can be found in an advertisement from 1784 promoting the spice and its availability at Sorlie's Perfumery Warehouse. Among the benefits of turmeric, the ad claimed, was that it "renders the stomach active in digestion—the blood naturally free in circulation—the mind vigorous—and contributes most of any food to an increase in the human race."

By the nineteenth century, the use of turmeric in recipes also began to appear in cookbooks written by authors in the United States. For example, a curry recipe calling for turmeric was included in the book *The Virginia Housewife; Or, Methodical Cook* authored by Mary Randolph (1762–1828) and published in 1824. Randolph's work was one of the most popular and influential books on cooking and housekeeping in America right up to the 1860s.

But it was not until the twentieth century that Western herbalists and scientists first began to truly investigate turmeric's medicinal properties. Research into its various benefits began in earnest in the West in the second half of the twentieth century, and has exploded during the last few decades. As a result, Western scientists have now verified many of the healing benefits offered by turmeric, many of which were first accounted for in Ayurveda and traditional Chinese medicine thousands of years ago. Based on this research, pharmaceutical companies are now exploring ways in which they can synthesize turmeric's active ingredients to develop potentially new drugs. In addition, various cosmetic firms are now using turmeric in their products, such as beauty creams and facial cleansing products. Clearly, at long last, Western science is beginning to catch up to their ancient counterparts in India and China.

TURMERIC'S NUTRITIONAL PROPERTIES

The reason why turmeric is being shown by scientific research to provide a wide range of benefits, in large part, has to do with the nutrients it contains. According to the national nutrient database of the United States Department of Agriculture (USDA), turmeric powder contains the following vitamins and minerals:

- calcium
- copper
- iron
- magnesium
- manganese
- phosphorus
- potassium
- sodium

- vitamin B_2 (riboflavin)
- vitamin B_3 (niacin)
- vitamin B_6 (pyridoxine)
- vitamin B_9 (folate)
- vitamin C
- vitamin E
- vitamin K
- zinc

Let's take a look at the various health benefits each of these nutrients provide.

Calcium

Calcium is best known for its importance in building and maintaining strong bones, teeth, and connective tissue, but it plays other important roles in the body, as well. Among them are aiding digestion by producing enzymes involved in the digestive process, assisting in healthy blood clotting, and regulating the nerve impulses that signal muscles, including muscles of the heart, to contract. Research indicates that calcium can also help prevent high blood pressure and may reduce the risk of developing colon cancer. Although calcium supplements are a popular way for people to ensure they meet their bodies' calcium needs, a growing body of evidence is showing that the best way to obtain calcium is through food.

Copper

Copper plays a variety of roles in the body, including helping to regulate and protect the cardiovascular and nervous systems. The body uses copper to produce superoxide dismutase (SOD). Found in all living cells, SOD acts as a powerful antioxidant that protects cells, tissues, and organs from free radical damage. Copper also plays a role in maintaining the health of skin and hair, and is used by the body to create melanin, the pigment that gives skin, hair, and eyes their color.

Copper is useful in maintaining bone health and the overall skeletal system, and helps protect against rheumatoid arthritis, osteoporosis, and joint pain. In addition, it is used to produce phospholipids, the substances that are a component of all cell membranes, and which form the myelin sheaths that cover and protect nerves. Copper is also necessary to protect against atherosclerosis and to prevent arteries from rupturing. It can help protect against aneurysms and heart arrhythmias, and is required for keeping blood properly oxygenated and regulating blood pressure levels.

Copper also assists in the production of hemoglobin in red blood cells. While iron itself is the primary producer of hemoglobin, copper supports the process by properly maintaining and releasing the body's iron stores when hemoglobin is produced. For this reason, copper supplementation is sometimes used to treat anemia in addition to iron.

Iron

Iron is required in the production of hemoglobin in red blood cells, and works synergistically with copper in this process. Hemoglobin transports oxygen throughout the body and gives red blood cells their color. Iron deficiencies can lead to anemia, a condition characterized by fatigue, shortness of breath, and pale skin caused by a lack of oxygen. Iron also helps supply muscles with oxygen so that they contract and function properly.

Magnesium

Magnesium is quite possibly the most important mineral required for optimal health. Primarily acting within the cells, magnesium is responsible for the proper functioning of approximately 80 percent of the body's metabolic processes. It does this by activating more than a thousand metabolic pathways in the body, including those responsible for protein, carbohydrate, and fat metabolism. Magnesium plays a vital role in energy metabolism because it is essential for the production and functioning of adenosine triphosphate (ATP), the cells' main source of energy generation. Magnesium is also the essential nutrient for muscles, playing a vital role in their proper functioning and, most importantly, their relaxation. Without magnesium, your muscles literally could not operate the way nature intended.

One of magnesium's most important functions is supporting the heart and overall cardiovascular system. Magnesium is absolutely vital for proper heart function, and plays a crucial role in protecting against heart disease, including heart attacks, stroke, and hypertension (high blood pressure).

Research shows that magnesium acts as a natural calcium channel blocker, but without any of the health risks posed by calcium channel blocker drugs, and also helps to prevent the formation of dangerous blood clots. And its role in ATP production is also essential for protecting the heart, since heart muscle cells contain very high concentrations of mitochondria that depend on ATP to do their job. In addition, magnesium helps dilate blood vessels, making it easier for the heart to pump blood and more effectively transmit nutrients and oxygen to the body's cells, tissues, and organs.

Among its many other functions, magnesium enhances immune function and helps protect against infection, copies and repairs DNA, and aids in proper cell division, maintenance, and repair. It also acts as a "gatekeeper" for the cells by modulating the electrical potential across cell membranes. This, in turn, enables nutrients to enter into cells and cellular waste products to be excreted. One of the primary ways in which magnesium helps to accomplish this task is by regulating the cells' sodium/potassium pump, an active transport system that is responsible for ensuring that cells contain relatively high concentrations of potassium ions but low concentrations of sodium ions. Maintaining healthy ratios of high potassium to low sodium ions within the cells and high sodium to low potassium ions outside the cells is important. When this ratio is disturbed, the stage is set for disease to occur at the cellular level of the body.

Magnesium protects against the accumulation of environmental toxins in the cells and tissues, and helps the body produce glutathione, a powerful antioxidant that protects against free radical damage and toxicity. It helps activate and regulate hormones, as well, including the support of proper functioning of the thyroid gland and other endocrine organs. It also regulates nerve function, and, along with calcium, is essential for healthy bones and teeth. And it prevents unhealthy calcium buildup (calcification) in the arteries and inside the kidneys, in addition to regulating blood sugar levels.

Manganese

Manganese acts as an antioxidant, helping to prevent free radical damage. It also plays a role in maintaining healthy digestion, and helps the body convert fats and protein into energy. In addition, manganese helps bones grow and stay healthy and is useful for preventing and relieving osteoporosis. Among its other functions are preventing and reducing fatigue levels, regulating blood sugar levels, and improving thyroid function.

Manganese also supports the immune, nervous, and reproductive systems. It plays a role in normal blood clotting and is needed for the body's production of cartilage and fluids in the joints that keep them lubricated.

Lastly, manganese helps the body absorb vitamin B_1 and vitamin E, and works with all B vitamins to help prevent and relieve anxiety, depression, and other nervous disorders.

Phosphorus

Phosphorus is found in every cell of the body, but is most abundant in bones and teeth, where it plays an essential role in their proper formation. It also helps the body metabolize carbohydrates and fats, and is involved in the growth, maintenance, and repair of cells and tissues. Like magnesium, phosphorus helps the body produce ATP, and, like manganese, it works synergistically with all B vitamins. It also supports a healthy heartbeat, kidney function, muscle contractions, and proper nerve signaling.

Potassium

Potassium is another vitally important mineral, and plays a key part of the cells' sodium/potassium pump. Potassium acts as an electrolyte, meaning that it helps electricity flow through your body. Most potassium in your body is found inside of your cells, but it moves outside of cell walls if necessary in order to keep fluid steady in and around cells. This process, known as *cellular membrane potential,* is heavily regulated by the body in order to govern and sustain healthy electrical flow for the rhythm of your heartbeat. In addition, potassium is required for healthy nerve and muscle function, and for maintaining proper blood pressure and blood sugar levels.

Lack of potassium in the body can result in a number of health problems, including a condition known as *hypokalemia,* which is caused when potassium is rapidly depleted from the body faster than it can be replenished, such as what happens with prolonged vomiting, diarrhea, and the overuse of diuretics. Symptoms of potassium deficiency include fatigue, muscle cramps, bloating, constipation, abdominal pain, acne, depression, edema, nervousness, insatiable thirst, high cholesterol, insomnia, nausea, problems breathing, and sodium (salt) retention.

Sodium

Sodium (salt) has been demonized in recent decades as something that should be avoided. In truth, however, sodium is another important electrolyte. It is vital for the health of the body's extracellular fluid, and is an essential part of the cells' sodium/potassium pump. Sodium also plays a crucial role in various enzyme functions in the body, and is required for regulating the body's other fluids. It supports healthy muscle contraction, as well as helps to maintain the cardiovascular and nervous systems. Without sodium, your body would not be able to properly generate and transmit electrical impulses. Sodium also supports the health of the adrenal glands, and aids in glucose absorption.

Your body's sodium stores can become depleted when you sweat profusely or stay out in the sun too long in hot weather. Signs of sodium deficiency include confusion, diarrhea, dizziness, fatigue, headache, low blood pressure, muscle pain, and weakness.

Vitamin B_2

Vitamin B_2, or riboflavin, plays a variety of important roles in the body. It regulates red blood cell growth and boosts immune function by protecting the body from free radical damage. Like B_1, B_2 is necessary for the conversion of food into energy. It does this by producing two enzymes, known, respectively, as flavin mononucleotide and flavin adenine dinucleotide, both of which are necessary to convert proteins, carbohydrates, and fats into energy.

B_2 is needed in order for other B vitamins, especially vitamins B_3 and B_6, to properly perform their functions. In addition, B_2 transforms vitamin B_5 and folic acid into neurotransmitters, which are crucial for healthy brain function. Lastly, B_2 is required to maintain the health of hair, nails, skin, and vision.

Vitamin B_3

Vitamin B_3, or niacin, works in conjunction with other B vitamins to produce and release energy in the cells, and to maintain proper functioning of the nervous system. It is also necessary to maintain proper circulation in the body, as well as regulating blood sugar levels and the production of hormones. Without B_3, the body cannot produce sufficient amounts of hydrochloric acid (HCl) in the stomach, which is essential for healthy digestion, especially of protein foods.

One of B_3's most important functions is its ability to maintain healthy levels of both HDL and LDL cholesterol. This fact was proven by research conducted in the 1950s by Drs. Abram Hoffer and Linus Pauling, who found that supplementation of vitamin B_3 boosted levels of HDL ("good") cholesterol while simultaneously lowering levels of LDL ("bad") cholesterol. Unlike cholesterol drugs, especially statin drugs, B_3 provides these important health benefits without causing any side effects.

Research has also shown that B_3 is helpful for preventing and treating a wide range of health conditions, ranging from canker sores, circulatory problems, depression, diarrhea, digestive problems, dizziness, fatigue, headache, inflammation, insomnia, low blood sugar, muscle cramps, PMS, Raynaud's disease, and tinnitus. It also helps to maintain healthy skin.

Vitamin B$_6$

Vitamin B$_6$, or pyridoxine, has many uses in the body. Among them are help-ing to convert foods into energy, boosting immune function, and maintaining the health of the nervous system. B$_6$ is also an essential nutrient for protect-ing against heart disease, due to its ability, in combination with vitamins B$_9$ (folate) and B$_{12}$, to prevent the formation of homocysteine, a common dietary amino acid which comes mostly from meat. Elevated levels of homocysteine are a major risk factor for atherosclerosis (hardening of the arteries), heart disease, and stroke because of how it attracts cholesterol and causes it to be deposited within the arteries and muscles of the heart. B$_6$ can also break down homocysteine after it forms.

B$_6$ helps prevent the formation of unhealthy blood clots that can trigger both heart attack and stroke. In addition, B$_6$ aids in maintaining healthy blood circulation and regulating hormone production. Finally, B$_6$ can help prevent and reverse varicose veins, and minimize symptoms of carpal tunnel syn-drome, diabetes, and PMS.

Vitamin B$_9$

Vitamin B$_9$, or folate, plays a crucial role for energy production, and is neces-sary for the overall health of all of the body's cells. It also plays a vital role in the body's growth processes, beginning with the development of the fetus, making it an essential vitamin for women during pregnancy and breastfeed-ing. In addition, B$_9$ helps boost immune function, regulates the production of both red and white blood cells, and is involved in the production of both DNA and RNA. It helps maintain the health of the gastrointestinal tract, as well as the skin, the cells that line the small intestine, and red and white blood cells. Folate also helps form the DNA and RNA in our genes, which are needed to regulate cell formation.

Vitamin C

Vitamin C is one of the most versatile and important nutrients that the body needs. Similarly to B vitamins, vitamin C is water-soluble. It cannot be pro-duced by the body and so must be replenished on a daily basis via diet and, if necessary, as a nutritional supplement.

One of the staunchest advocates for vitamin C was the late Linus Pauling, PhD, who touted its health benefits beginning in the 1950s and throughout the rest of his life. Despite having won both the Nobel Prize for Science and the Nobel Peace Prize, and being ranked as one of the top twenty scientists of all time, Dr. Pauling's views about vitamin C were dismissed as "quackery" by the medical establishment right up until his death in 1994, at age ninety-three.

Only later did most of his claims about vitamin C become widely accepted, just as he assured me they would be when I had the great privilege of being able to interview Dr. Pauling at length by telephone in 1992.

Dr. Pauling believed that daily supplementation with enough vitamin C could potentially prolong one's life by as much as twelve to eighteen years. Given how important it is to so many processes in the body, it is easy to understand his viewpoint. Vitamin C is one of the most powerful antioxidants among all nutrients, and is essential for maintaining healthy tissues, repairing damaged tissues, protecting against cancer, and boosting overall immune function. It also plays a vital role in protecting the heart and overall cardiovascular system, maintaining optimal levels of collagen in the skin, and ensuring the health of bones, gums, and teeth. It is necessary for preventing supplies of folic acid from being broken down too quickly in the body, thus improving its absorption and usefulness. It is also required for the body to properly absorb and use iron.

Vitamin C also acts as a potent anti-inflammatory agent, thereby protecting and helping to reverse a wide range of health conditions associated with chronic inflammation, including allergies, arthritis, bronchitis and other respiratory conditions, bruising, diabetes, fatigue, fibromyalgia, joint pain, and sprains. In addition, research shows that vitamin C helps maintain the health of the eyes, and can prevent cataracts, eyestrain, glaucoma, and other vision problems. It has also been shown to be helpful for preventing and relieving constipation, hangover, infertility, rashes, shingles, skin wrinkling, and sunburn. Because of its strong anti-bacterial and anti-viral properties, vitamin C is an important nutrient for preventing and combating a wide range of infectious diseases, ranging from colds and flu to gastrointestinal infections, yeast infections, and urinary tract infections.

Vitamin E

Vitamin E is another important antioxidant that neutralizes free-radical damage. It is also a powerful immune-enhancing nutrient. Like vitamin C, vitamin E plays a crucial role in protecting the immune system, primarily because of its ability to increase levels of the interferon and interleukin, two biochemicals that are required by the immune system to prevent and fight off infections. Research has shown that adequate vitamin E levels in the body can help protect against a variety of other conditions as well, including certain types of cancer, respiratory conditions, various eye problems, including macular degeneration and vision issues related to diabetes, prostate enlargement, osteoarthritis, and sunburn. It has also shown promise for preventing Alzheimer's disease and dementia.

Vitamin K

Vitamin K plays a variety of important roles in the body. One of the most vital has to do with its ability to produce various blood-clotting factors in the body that are essential to prevent unchecked bleeding or hemorrhaging. Vitamin K is also necessary to maintain the health of the capillaries. It helps to protect against and heal bruises and nosebleeds, as well.

In addition, it keeps bones strong and healthy by enhancing their ability to absorb and store calcium. Studies have shown that lack of vitamin K can increase the risk of bone diseases such as osteoporosis, while also reducing the risks of bone and hip fractures. In part, this is due to how vitamin K interacts and works with vitamin D. It also prevents vitamin D from causing excess calcium to be displaced into the arteries and kidneys, thus reducing the risk of atherosclerosis and kidney stones, as well as other types of kidney disease associated with excess calcium buildup. Recently, researchers have also begin to study vitamin K's potential for reducing the risk of cancerous tumors.

Zinc

Zinc is another important mineral with many important functions in the body. Not only does zinc act as a potent antioxidant, it is also necessary for the health of both the thymus gland and the immune system, especially with regard to the production of T-cells. It enhances digestion, helps maintain the health of the reproductive system (especially in men, due to its ability to boost the production of growth hormones and testosterone), and is needed for healthy bones, hair, skin, and nails. Additionally, zinc helps maintain the health of the eyes (especially the retina) and ears, and can help prevent tinnitus. It also boosts the effectiveness of vitamin A.

Research has shown that zinc can be effective in preventing and relieving a variety of health conditions, including acne, arthritis, colds and flu, canker sores, fibromyalgia, hemorrhoids, lupus, macular degeneration, and sore throat. It also speeds wound healing and can be an effective treatment for various other skin conditions, such as eczema, rosacea, and psoriasis.

Beneficial as the above nutrients are to your health, their inclusion in turmeric is not enough to fully explain how and why turmeric is such a healthy spice. Certainly, all of these nutrients provide part of the answer to such questions. But the full answer also lies with another important ingredient that turmeric powder contains. I'm referring to *curcumin*, the ingredient that gives turmeric its characteristic bright yellowish-orange color.

CURCUMIN'S POTENT HEALTH PROPERTIES

Curcumin is the primary active ingredient in turmeric, part of a family of active compounds known as *curcuminoids.* It is found in the root of the turmeric plant and, as mentioned, is what gives the spice its distinctive color.

Curcumin belongs to a class of nutrients known as *polyphenols.* Phenols are organic compounds that act as one of nature's basic chemical building blocks. Polyphenols get their name because they contain more than one phenol group per molecule—the term polyphenol literally means "more than one phenol." They are the most abundant class of phenol compounds found in all plants and are part of a larger group of compounds known as antioxidants, which act to prevent your body's cells and tissues from becoming damaged because of oxidation, a process in which cells and tissues literally begin to "rust out." So far, scientists have identified over 8,000 different types of polyphenols in plants.

Polyphenols are responsible for many plant qualities, including their color, flavor, scent, and taste. They also help to keep plants strong and healthy by protecting them from harmful bacteria and fungi, as well as from insects and ultraviolet light. Over the last few decades, research has found that polyphenols are also responsible for many of the health-promoting properties that fruits, vegetables, nuts, seeds, and grains provide us when we eat them.

One of the main reasons why polyphenols are so important to good health is because they act as catalysts that enable other nutrients to properly do their job. Additionally, unlike most other nutrients, the health benefits polyphenols, including curcumin, provide are very broad in scope, enabling them to simultaneously regulate a wide variety of different cell functions. By contrast, nutrients such as vitamins, although they are also vital for good health, typically serve very specific and limited functions in cellular metabolism.

As research into the healing properties of turmeric continues, it is becoming increasingly evident that it is curcumin, far more so than the various other nutrients that turmeric contains, that is primarily responsible for the health benefits the plant can provide. For this reason, more and more research studies today are focused on curcumin extracts alone, rather than turmeric itself.

Based on these studies, scientists have confirmed that curcumin acts as a potent antioxidant, making it an effective natural aid in preventing against and reversing free radical damage in the body's cells, tissues, and organs. Free radical damage is a major contributor to a wide range of degenerative disease conditions, as well as premature aging.

Research also shows that curcumin has powerful anti-inflammatory properties. Additionally, it is a natural analgesic (pain reliever), and shows great promise as an anticancer and anti-tumor agent. It also has the ability to protect against bacteria, viruses, and other harmful microbes due to its ability to enhance immune function.

Other research has confirmed that curcumin, unlike most natural substances, is capable of crossing the blood-brain barrier. This protective membrane is designed to prevent toxins, infectious bacteria and viruses, and other harmful substances from penetrating and affecting the brain. However, the blood-brain barrier can also prevent various nutrients from reaching the brain. This is not the case with curcumin. As a result, it is able to deliver its antioxidant and anti-inflammatory benefits directly to brain tissue, making it a vital natural aid in protecting against Alzheimer's disease, dementia, depression, and other brain diseases that are known to be caused and exacerbated by free radicals and chronic inflammation.

All told, curcumin's healing properties explain why both it and turmeric continue to gain a reputation as natural healing agents for a wide range of diseases. That's because nearly all chronic conditions are caused by the very factors that curcumin and turmeric both protect against (free radical damage, infections, inflammation, pain, and cancer cell and tumor growth). In the rest of the book, you will learn more about turmeric's and curcumin's proven benefits for the most serious of these diseases.

CONCLUSION

Having read this far, you now know how and why turmeric has been used for thousands of years in India, China, and other Asian countries, not only as a dye and flavoring agent, but also as a medicinal spice. You also learned that over the past few decades, modern science has begun to catch up with what practitioners of both Ayurveda and traditional Chinese medicine have known about turmeric's healing properties for centuries. Not only have Western scientists confirmed many of the health benefits attributed to turmeric by both systems of Eastern medicine, they have also discovered that it is turmeric's active ingredient, curcumin, that is largely responsible for its health-enhancing properties.

In Chapter 2, you will discover how and why both turmeric and curcumin can help protect you against one of the primary underlying causes of most of today's chronic, serious diseases: inflammation.

2

How Turmeric Protects
Against Inflammation

Although you likely don't realize it right now, as you read these words, chances are high that the inside of your body is on fire. The fire I'm referring to is inflammation.

Under normal, healthy circumstances, inflammation acts as a natural healing mechanism in the body. Under such circumstances, inflammation is short-lived and acts as an essential immune response. Without it, your body could not heal wounds, burns, or other injuries, nor could it protect you from harmful, invading bacteria, viruses, or other microorganisms.

This type of inflammation response is known as *acute inflammation*. When it occurs, a variety of reactions in your body are set in motion. Should you cut your finger, for example, your body's immune system will cause blood cells, proteins, and other compounds to swarm around the cut in order to begin the healing process. As this happens, the affected area in your finger will turn red and likely swell as blood clots form around the cut in an effort to stop the bleeding. As healing proceeds, the inflammatory response will subside and eventually be completely deactivated once the cut is fully healed.

A similar response occurs whenever your body successfully fights off invading microorganisms. In such cases, your immune system will again trigger various compounds, as well as immune cells, to surround and engulf these invaders and prevent them from spreading further. This acute inflammation response keeps the invaders at bay, enabling the immune cells to destroy and eliminate them.

Based on the above examples, you can see why an acute inflammation response is both beneficial and necessary for continued good health. However, when the inflammation response becomes chronic, meaning when it does not subside as nature intended, it sets the stage for a wide variety of health problems to occur, including today's most serious diseases, such as Alzheimer's and dementia, cancer, and heart disease.

From the perspective of conventional medicine, chronic inflammation typically occurs when an acute inflammation response fails to heal or resolve an injury or infection, at which point medical intervention is often necessary. However, chronic inflammation can also occur in the absence of injury or infection. When it does so, it is almost always due to a variety of other factors, all of which act as stressors in the body that trigger an ongoing inflammation response.

Very often, in such cases, chronic inflammation escapes detection or is ignored by doctors until it progresses to the point where it manifests as a disease condition. In the meantime, the compounds and immune cells that play a role in the acute inflammation process can start to change, becoming harmful and capable of causing ongoing damage to previously healthy organs and tissues in your body. Because chronic inflammation usually does not present with the obvious symptoms characteristic of acute inflammation, it can be difficult to diagnose, yet its harmful effects can be quite powerful and, in some cases, even life-threatening. In fact, according to the Centers for Disease Control and Prevention, of the ten leading causes of death by disease in the United States, *chronic low-level inflammation* contributes to the onset and progression of at least seven such conditions: heart disease, cancer, chronic lower respiratory disease, stroke, Alzheimer's disease, diabetes, and nephritis (kidney disease).

As I wrote at the beginning of this chapter, due to a variety of factors that are so common in our modern, stress-filled world, it is quite likely that this process of chronic inflammation, to some degree, is taking place inside you right now. Fortunately, there is quite a lot you can do on your own to put a stop to it, including using turmeric, as I explain below. First, let's take a closer look at the many disease conditions that are now linked to chronic inflammation.

THE WIDE RANGE OF DISEASES CAUSED BY CHRONIC INFLAMMATION

The range of disease conditions caused by inflammation continues to expand as scientists and physicians progress in their understanding of how chronic low-grade (non-acute) inflammation triggers illness in the body. In addition to chronic pain, research has now established that chronic inflammation plays a primary role in nearly all degenerative diseases, including Alzheimer's and dementia, cancer, type 2 (adult-onset) diabetes, fibromyalgia, heart disease, migraine headache, multiple sclerosis (MS), Parkinson's disease, and stroke.

Inflammation has also been implicated in a long list of conditions, including:

- ADD/ADHD
- allergies
- asthma
- autism
- carpal tunnel syndrome
- Celiac and Crohn's disease
- chronic fatigue
- dental issues
- gallbladder disease
- GERD and other gastrointestinal problems

- Guillain-Barre disease
- eczema
- fibrosis
- kidney disease and kidney failure
- liver disease
- lupus
- neuropathy
- obesity
- psoriasis
- thyroid problems

In addition, essentially any disease that ends in *-itis* is caused by chronic inflammation. This includes such conditions such as ankylosing spondylitis, arthritis, bronchitis, bursitis, colitis, gastritis, pancreatitis, and tendonitis. Even such conditions such as anxiety and depression, which until recently were considered mental/emotional issues, have now been linked to chronic inflammation.

All told, chronic inflammation is the likely cause of virtually all chronic disease conditions, each of which is classified by conventional medicine as a specific illness that is not related to other conditions. In reality, however, they *are* related because of the fact that they all result from the same underlying cause: an overactive and ongoing inflammatory response in the body. In most cases, the type of disease that develops simply depends upon which organ system in the body happens to be most susceptible to the cascade of unhealthy processes that chronic inflammation triggers.

Given everything that scientists and physicians have discovered about the primary role chronic inflammation plays in such a wide range of serious disease conditions, clearly preventing and reversing inflammation is of paramount importance in also preventing and reversing the diseases themselves. Simply put, *unless and until chronic inflammation is properly dealt with and eliminated, the diseases it can cause cannot and will not be healed.*

At best, all that will be achieved is a managing of symptoms, which is precisely what most conventional physicians seek to do, usually relying on pharmaceutical drugs that do not address the real cause of the diseases—inflammation—and also carry a high risk of serious side effects. This limited and very often futile approach is one of the main reasons why health care costs in the United States continue to skyrocket (currently over $3 trillion a year), while the incidence of chronic, degenerative diseases also continues to climb.

RISK FACTORS THAT CAUSE CHRONIC INFLAMMATION

At its heart, chronic inflammation is synonymous with the human body's immune system being locked into an "on" position, meaning that it continues to operate as if the body is facing harmful infections or has been injured in some way, when in actuality neither of those issues is usually present (in some cases, allergens and harmful microorganisms that have escaped conventional diagnostic techniques and other detection methods may be present in the body).

So, what are the factors that cause the immune system to become "stuck" in this "on" position? It turns out that there are a variety of factors responsible for this.

Diet

Most of the risk factors for chronic inflammation originate in or affect your gut. This is not surprising, since research continues to establish how closely interrelated immune function is to the health of the body's overall gastrointestinal system. Simply put, suboptimal gastrointestinal function results in diminished immune function, while simultaneously triggering and maintaining the body's inflammation response.

Given that fact, the most common factors that result in chronic inflammation are related to your diet. This especially true of diets that include excess amounts of sugars and carbohydrates (particularly simple, or "white" carbohydrates such as breads, pastas, and white rice); foods containing transfatty acids; excessive amounts of unsaturated and polyunsaturated vegetable oils; excessive intake of meats, dairy products, and other foods that have an acidifying effect in the body once they are metabolized; consumption of fast, or "junk," foods; and a lack of healthy saturated fats and fresh fruits and vegetables. Inadequate water intake throughout the day can also cause chronic inflammation, or make it worse, as can an excessive consumption of grains.

Eating fried or barbequed foods or foods that are overly cooked is also a common cause of chronic inflammation, as such foods, when consumed,

The Vicious Cycle of "Fire" and "Rust"

Inflammation can be likened to fire within the body, while oxidation, if excessive, can cause tissues and organs to "rust," in the same way that an apple, when cut and exposed to air, rapidly begins to turn brown as it comes in contact with the oxygen the air contains. Research has shown that chronic inflammation and oxidation feed into each other, creating a vicious cycle of harmful health consequences.

In the body, oxidation occurs when atoms lose an electron. These missing electrons are replaced by substances known as free radicals. Free radical damage is a major health risk, which is why antioxidant foods and nutritional supplements are so often recommended by nutritionally oriented physicians. (Antioxidants "quench" free radicals, helping to prevent damage to the body's cells, tissues, and organs caused by oxidative stress.)

Both a certain degree of inflammation and oxidation in the body is necessary for good health, however. Your body's inflammatory response is one of the ways in which it acts to protect and heal itself from injury, trauma, and infection, for example. And without enough oxygen in your blood, you would very quickly become sick and might even die, which is why today growing numbers of doctors are turning to oxidative therapies that improve the body's internal oxygen supply to treat serious infections, as well as, in some cases, cancer, heart disease, stroke, and other serious conditions. However, prolonged or chronic inflammation in the body is dangerous, as is excessive levels of oxidation, and both are now known to be primary causes of a wide range of diseases.

unleash what are known as *advanced glycation end products* (AGEs) into the bloodstream. AGEs are formed by an unhealthy binding of sugars with proteins and fats. In addition to triggering inflammation in the body, they also generate free radicals, which cause damage due to their oxidative effects on the body's tissues and organs.

Excessive consumption of food, and therefore calories, can also trigger or exacerbate chronic inflammation. A number of studies have shown that when individuals follow calorie-restrictive diets, they can significantly reduce their risk of developing chronic inflammation, and also reverse it.

High Blood Sugar

High blood sugar is another major risk factor for chronic inflammation. The reason for this is because of how excess glucose (sugar) in the bloodstream fuels inflammation in the body. Because the standard American diet (rightly known as SAD) is high in sugars, simple carbohydrates, and other glucose-rich foods and beverages (soda, commercial fruit juice, etc.), high blood pressure, also known as *hypoglycemia,* is an increasingly common health problem in the United States.

Glucose is the primary energy source used by the body's cells to produce and utilize energy. However, excess glucose that is not used to produce energy is converted by the body into triglycerides and then stored as fat. It also accumulates in the bloodstream, causing high blood sugar. Not only do glucose-derived triglycerides in the bloodstream contribute to the formation of plaque in the arteries that cause atherosclerosis, heart disease, and stroke, they also act as a trigger for both chronic inflammation and oxidation. In addition, excess glucose in the body negatively interacts with various proteins in the body to cause glycation reactions, further fueling chronic inflammation and the production of harmful free radicals.

You can easily be tested for high blood sugar by asking your doctor to conduct a fasting blood glucose test. The test is very simple and only requires a drop of your blood obtained via a pinprick. Before it is administered, you will need to avoid eating or consuming any beverages aside from water for a period of at least eight hours, which is why the test is most often administered in the morning before a person eats that day. According to conventional medicine, a fasting glucose level below 100 mg/dL indicates that you do not have high blood sugar. However, a growing number of physicians and researchers now view fasting glucose levels between 70 and 85 mg/dL to be a far more optimal range. This range can usually be achieved by avoiding sugar and limiting your intake of all carbohydrate foods (both simple and complex).

Hormone Imbalances

Hormone imbalances, especially a deficit of sex hormones in the body, are another significant contributor to chronic inflammation. Sex hormones (estrogen, progesterone, and testosterone), play many important roles in the body, including helping to regulate both its immune and inflammatory responses. Immunity and inflammation are closely linked, with healthy, acute inflammatory responses being one of the major ways that your body's immune system deals with infections and wounds. Specific types of immune cells, such as macrophages and neutrophils, help to regulate your body's inflammation responses. Both types of cells also contain receptor sites for sex hormones, allowing them to appropriately respond to the level of sex hormones found in the body's various tissues.

Telltale Signs of Chronic Inflammation

Given that chronic inflammation often goes undetected even by many physicians until it progresses to a serious disease state, knowing and paying attention to the signs and symptoms of chronic inflammation is an important step you can take to safeguard your own health.

Three of the most common telltale signs are as follows:

Depression, Lack of Enthusiasm About Life

A growing body of scientific research is finding that markers of inflammation in the body are often elevated in people who suffer from depression, anxiety, or a diminished enthusiasm for life. Researchers in this area caution that not all cases of such conditions are caused by inflammation, either directly or indirectly, yet inflammation does appear to often be present in many instances. In addition, research has also shown that when inflammation is artificially induced in patients by medical means, feelings of anxiety and depression, as well as fatigue, typically soon follow. This is true even in tests in which inflammation was only mildly increased. Conversely, research has also shown that the use of anti-inflammatory nutrients and herbs, including turmeric and curcumin, can reduce feelings of depression as they work to also reduce inflammation.

Other signs that you may be unknowingly beset by chronic inflammation include:

- increased susceptibility to infectious diseases
- joint pain and stiffness
- persistent high blood pressure
- recurring acid reflux
- recurring urinary tract infections
- wrinkled skin and various other skin conditions

None of the above symptoms can be relied upon as definite diagnoses of chronic inflammation, especially since they can also be caused by a variety of other factors. But if you are affected by any of them, be sure to seek prompt medical attention and consult with your physician to determine the cause.

Lingering Fatigue

If you find yourself battling fatigue on a regular basis, despite getting enough sleep, eating right, and getting adequate exercise, undiagnosed chronic fatigue may be the underlying cause. That's because of how inflammation can affect your body's central nervous system (CNS), which includes your brain and spinal cord. With regard to fatigue, this is especially true for how inflammation can throw off the part of your brain that is responsible for regulating your body's responses to the circadian rhythm during both daylight and nighttime hours.

Research has shown that inflammation can significantly impair how this area of the brain, sometimes referred to as a "circadian pacemaker," functions, leading to ongoing experiences of fatigue and sluggishness. Some researchers, including Mary Harrington, PhD, director of the neuroscience program at Smith College, in Northampton, Massachusetts, estimate that as much as 15 percent of the United States population is coping with lingering fatigue due to how chronic inflammation is affecting this area of the brain.

Stomach Upset or Pain

As I mentioned earlier in this chapter, poor diet and impaired gastrointestinal function are leading causes of chronic inflammation in the body, and the stomach and overall GI tract are some of the first areas affected by chronic inflammation. If you suffer from ongoing or recurrent bouts of stomach upset or pain, as well as other persistent gastrointestinal problems, it is highly likely that chronic inflammation is the cause or a significant co-factor.

An adequate, balanced supply of sex hormones is necessary for the body's inflammation response to be properly regulated. As the supply of these hormones decline, however, the production of pro-inflammatory cytokines and other compounds can become unchecked. Research, for example, has found that as testosterone levels in men decline, there is an increase in pro-inflammatory cytokines. Studies have also shown that a similar increase in these cytokines occurs when estrogen production in women declines due to menopause, surgeries such as hysterectomy, and other factors. In addition, research shows that there is a spike in the incidence of numerous degenerative diseases that are known to be caused by chronic inflammation among men and women as they age past their prime, and the body's production of sex hormones declines.

In addition to the above factors, chronic inflammation is, for many, also a consequence of the aging process. When we are young and healthy, our bodies typically only increase their production of pro-inflammatory cytokines when we are exposed to infection or are injured. But in older men and women, even when they are otherwise healthy, very often markers for chronic inflammation, such as TNF-α and IL-06, are found to be elevated, according to research. This fact makes it all the more important that you do everything you can to prevent chronic inflammation from taking hold in your body, and to reverse it if it is already present, especially as you grow older.

Obesity

Being unhealthily overweight or obese is another significant cause of chronic inflammation. In addition, chronic inflammation can also trigger unhealthy weight gain, creating a vicious cycle between these two major detriments to your health.

Unhealthy weight results in an increase of fat tissues in the body. These tissues act in much the same way that endocrine (hormone) glands do, both producing and storing various hormones, as well as a special class of proteins called *cytokines,* which help regulate the body's inflammatory response. Among these cytokines produced by fat tissues are TNF-α and IL-6, both of which are known to trigger strong inflammatory responses in the body, and have been linked by research to chronic inflammation. TNF-α has also been linked to cancer.

Excess abdominal fat (also known as visceral fat) caused by obesity is a particularly dangerous risk factor for chronic inflammation, because it is within this layer of fat that TNF-α and IL-6 are produced in the highest amounts. Research has shown that abdominal fat cells and tissues can produce up to three times as much of these cytokines as other fat cells and tissues in the body. Additional research has also found that, in people who are overweight, abdominal fat cells and tissues cause as much as 35 percent of the body's total IL-6 production.

Further compounding this problem is the fact that in obese individuals, immune cells known as *macrophages* can infiltrate fat tissues, where they then secrete a variety of inflammation-causing cytokines. The accumulation of macrophages within fat tissue has been shown to be in direct proportion to a person's body mass index (BMI), a commonly used measurement of obesity and excess weight gain. The greater a person's BMI, the greater the accumulation of macrophages found in fat tissue. Research has shown the infiltration of macrophages in fat tissues is a primary cause of chronic inflammation, as well as insulin resistance, in people who are unhealthily overweight or obese.

Poor Sleep

According to national surveys, the inability to get a good night's sleep is affecting greater numbers of Americans every year, with insomnia and other sleeping problems becoming increasingly common. Research now shows that lack of healthy sleep is another causative factor of chronic inflammation. This is not surprising when we consider that the body's production of various pro-inflammatory cytokines follow its natural circadian rhythm (the twenty-four hour period of waking and sleeping).

Studies now indicate that these cytokines are likely involved in the regulation of sleep in both humans and animals. Additional research has shown that poor sleep results in an elevated production of these cytokines, as well as stress-related, pro-inflammatory hormones, regardless of a person's age or body mass index. Therefore, getting a good night's sleep is another crucial step in the battle against chronic inflammation.

Stress

Chronic stress can also cause or perpetuate chronic inflammation. This is the case regardless of the type of stress you may be under: physical, environmental, emotional, or mental. In response to stress, your body secretes various pro-inflammatory cytokines and stress hormones, such as cortisol, which have also been linked to chronic inflammation.

Chronic stress is also associated with poor sleep and excessive weight gain, both of which are also major contributors of chronic inflammation. In sum, the degree and frequency of the stress you experience in your daily life can have a significant impact on the degree of chronic inflammation your body develops.

Smoking

It's well-known that smoking is one of the leading causes of serious disease, most especially cancer and heart disease. One of the reasons this is so is because smoking cigarettes exposes the body to a variety of inflammation-triggering substances, including reactive oxygen species (ROS). ROS are highly reactive molecules. Though they are also produced in the body under normal, healthy circumstances, when left unchecked or introduced into the body from smoking, they can cause free radical damage because of the unpaired electrons they contain. This, in turn, can cause chronic inflammation.

Smoking also results in an increased production of multiple pro-inflammatory cytokines, while simultaneously interfering with and reducing the body's ability to produce its various anti-inflammatory compounds. Smoking also increases the risk of gum, or periodontal disease, which is now recognized as another major risk factor for chronic inflammation.

WORKING WITH YOUR DOCTOR
TO SCREEN FOR CHRONIC INFLAMMATION

Knowing whether or not you are afflicted by chronic inflammation is a crucial step in assessing your overall health. However, because many doctors do not screen their patients for chronic inflammation unless they are specifically asked by them to do so, don't hesitate to ask your own physician to provide such screening for you and your loved ones.

Screening for chronic inflammation can be done by using blood tests. The two most common blood tests used for this purpose are both inexpensive and measure the amount of pro-inflammatory markers in the bloodstream. These markers are *high sensitivity C-reactive protein,* or hs-CRP, and *fibrinogen.* Both these markers can be used to detect chronic inflammation and also to monitor your progress as you and your doctor work to reduce inflammation levels in your body. The hs-CRP test can also be used to determine your risk of heart disease and stroke. Any hs-CRP reading above 3.0 mg/L is an indication of chronic inflammation. The higher the reading, the more likely it is that systemic chronic inflammation is present. The optimal hs-CRP level for men is anything under 0.55 mg/L, while for women it should be under 1.5 mg/L.

Fibrinogen is a type of protein that acts as a blood clotting agent in the body. Like CRP, it is also a useful marker for determining the presence of chronic inflammation. In both men and women, the optimal fibrinogen level is between 295 and 370 mg/dL.

If chronic inflammation is shown by the two blood tests above, it may be necessary to conduct additional tests in order to better determine the specific factors that are causing it. These tests can be expensive and involve testing for various cytokine levels in the blood. The cytokines most commonly tested for determining the various factors that may be causing systemic chronic inflammation are TNF-α and IL-6. Levels of two additional cytokines, Il-1 beta and IL-8, might also be tested. The healthy, normal range for TNF-α is any reading below 8.1 pg/mL. Healthy ranges for IL-6 are reading between 2—29 pg/mL. Healthy ranges for IL-1 beta, and IL-8 are readings below 15.0 pg/mL and 32.0 pg/mL respectively.

TURMERIC AND CURCUMIN HELP
REDUCE/PREVENT CHRONIC INFLAMMATION

Now that you have a better understanding of how and why chronic inflammation is such a serious risk factor for your health, let's examine how turmeric and its key ingredient, curcumin, can go a long way to protect you from this major health scourge.

The Link Between Anger
and Chronic Inflammation

Researchers have discovered that chronic inflammation not only poses a significant risk to one's physical well-being, it may also be responsible for triggering anger and violent behavior. These findings build on previous research that has established that chronic inflammation is implicated in as much as 15 percent of all cases of depression.

Animal studies have shown that introducing cytokine inflammatory proteins into the brains of cats and mice can cause an increase their aggressive behavior. The results of those tests led researchers to consider whether inflammation can have a similar effect in humans. In one such test, researchers measured the levels of C-reactive protein (CRP) and interleukin-6 (IL-6) in the blood of seventy people previously diagnosed with intermittent explosive disorder (IED), a condition characterized by repeated and impulsive acts of aggression, such as outbursts of anger, domestic abuse, road rage, and the destruction of property. The study also included sixty-one people diagnosed with non-aggression related psychiatric disorders, and a group of sixty-seven participants with no history of psychiatric problems. These latter two groups acted as controls for the study.

The results of the study established a direct relationship between elevated levels of CRP and IL-6 and aggressive acts and emotions in the IED group, but not in the control groups. These results remained consistent even after the researchers took into account and controlled for lifestyle factors and other differences between all three groups in the study. The study also found that both pro-inflammation markers were especially elevated in people who had a history of more aggressive behaviors in the past.

Commenting of the study's findings, one of its lead researchers, Dr. Emil Coccaro, professor of psychiatry at the University of Chicago, said, "We don't know yet if the inflammation triggers aggression, or aggressive feelings set off inflammation, but it's a powerful indication that the two are biologically connected, and a damaging combination." He added that the study's results opened new directions for additional research to determine whether or not reducing inflammation levels in people could lead to a corresponding reduction in aggressive behaviors.

Chances are, if you went to your doctor because of an inflammatory condition such as arthritis or joint pain, you would likely leave with a prescription for a non-steroidal anti-inflammatory drug (NSAID, such as ibuprofen or naproxen) or a glucocorticoid medication, such as hydrocortisone or prednisone. There are a number of shortcomings and problems with this approach. First, such drugs target only limited aspects of the body's overall chronic inflammatory response that we discussed previously, leaving the other factors unchecked. Second, drug treatments alone cannot cure chronic inflammation. At best, they only provide relief from some of the symptoms caused by chronic inflammation. Third, and perhaps most importantly, all the pharmaceutical drugs that may be prescribed for inflammation are not meant for long-term use and can cause serious negative side effects that can make your health even worse.

While turmeric and curcumin are also not a cure, per se, for chronic inflammation, research has shown that they both can significantly reduce symptoms of inflammation. More significantly, unlike drugs, they can also prevent chronic inflammation from occurring in the first place. And they address far more of the causative factors that are involved in the inflammatory process than drugs do because of the broad spectrum of anti-inflammatory benefits they provide. Best of all, they do so with no risk of harmful side effects, and at a significantly lower financial cost.

A number of research studies have demonstrated that turmeric and curcumin can reduce and prevent the symptoms of chronic inflammation because of how they are able to target and block the multiple pathways of the body's inflammation signaling process. By doing so, both turmeric and curcumin are also able to protect against common diseases associated with chronic inflammation, including Alzheimer's disease and dementia, cancer, and heart disease. Moreover, in some cases, noticeable improvements in symptoms of chronic inflammation can occur within weeks, without any risk of negative side effects.

To further understand why turmeric and curcumin can provide superior benefits for people suffering from chronic inflammation than conventional medications can, let's take a closer look at how anti-inflammatory drugs work and contrast that with turmeric's and curcumin's mechanisms of action.

One of the most commonly prescribed classes of anti-inflammatory drugs are NSAIDs. They work primarily by acting as COX-1 and COX-2 inhibitors. Both COX-1 and COX-2 are types of enzymes called *cyclooxygenases* that produce prostaglandin-signaling molecules in the body. *Prostaglandins* are lipids (fats) that are involved in the body's inflammation response. Under normal circumstances, they play a role in the swelling, pain, and other temporary symptoms of acute inflammation, but also trigger these same symptoms on an ongoing basis during cases of chronic inflammation. By inhibiting COX-1 and COX-2, NSAIDs can help interrupt this particular inflammation pathway. But NSAIDs are not designed or intended for long-term use. Moreover, they can cause or contribute to other serious health problems, including liver damage, peptic ulcers, nausea, dizziness, constipation or diarrhea, extreme fatigue and weakness, and hearing problems, among other issues.

Turmeric and curcumin pose no such risks and can safely be consumed indefinitely, as turmeric's status as a staple spice in food dishes that are consumed on a daily basis in India and other lands where it is regularly used makes clear. Moreover, both turmeric and its key ingredient do far more than merely inhibit COX-1 and COX-2.

Researchers have long known that chronic inflammation in the body is caused and perpetuated by far more than prostaglandin-signaling molecules. For example, leukotriene-signaling molecules are also involved. *Leukotrienes* are a class of essential fatty acid metabolites (substances produced when the fatty acids are metabolized) that are precursors to prostaglandins. Just as prostaglandins are activated, in part, by the COX enzymes, leukotrienes are activated by an enzyme class known as LOX (lysyl oxidase). Scientists have shown that both turmeric and curcumin inhibit LOX enzymes just as they do COX enzymes. As a result, they are effective for inhibiting the multiple steps that occur in both prostaglandin and leukotriene production, thus providing broad-spectrum protection against chronic inflammation. This dual action is something that no class of anti-inflammatory drugs can do.

The ability of both turmeric and curcumin to inhibit LOX enzymes is vitally important for reasons far beyond chronic inflammation alone. As you will discover in more detail in Chapter 4, these enzymes have recently been discovered to play a vital role in enabling cancers to metastasize (spread). Approximately 90 percent of all deaths due to cancer occur as a direct result of metastasis. This is one of the reasons why turmeric and, especially, curcumin, play such an important role in protecting against cancer.

In addition to inhibiting both the COX and LOX enzymes that are involved in chronic inflammation, turmeric and curcumin provide anti-inflammatory mechanisms as well. *Inducible nitric oxide,* or iNOS, acts as a pro-inflammatory enzyme, similar to COX and LOX enzymes. It is involved in both acute (short-term) and chronic inflammation. In the latter type, it stimulates the production of pro-inflammatory cytokines. Inhibiting iNOS is yet another way by which turmeric and curcumin can help prevent and relieve symptoms of chronic inflammation. Similar benefits are also achieved by the ability of these compounds to inhibit NF-kappaB, which can also stimulate pro-inflammatory cytokines, and to regulate the production of prostaglandin E2 (PGE2) so that it is not produced in excessive amounts.

There is also another significant way that both turmeric and curcumin act as natural healers for chronic inflammation. This has to do with their potent antioxidant properties. Chronic inflammation and oxidation are inextricably linked, creating a vicious cycle with one another. Turmeric and curcumin help to arrest this cycle both by preventing and reducing chronic inflammation, and by also scavenging and eliminating free radicals that cause oxidation, such as hydroxyl radicals and superoxide. In addition, they also reduce the oxidation of fats and fatty acids in the body. Turmeric and curcumin have also been shown to reduce the likelihood that LDL, or "bad" cholesterol, becomes oxidized. As you will learn in Chapter 5, when it comes to heart disease, it is not elevated levels of LDL cholesterol that matters as much as whether or not the LDL cholesterol is oxidized.

Finally, both turmeric and curcumin have the ability to suppress the activation of macrophage immune cells and their migration to sites of inflammation in the body. Macrophages contribute to chronic inflammation. This fact has been borne out by a number of research studies. In one study, curcumin administered orally to mice resulted in reduced levels of a specific protein known as *macrophage recruiting factor monocyte chemoattractant protein 1*, or MCP-1, which activates macrophages and causes them to migrate to areas of the body susceptible to inflammation. It was also found that curcumin reduced levels of blood monocytes, from which macrophages are formed.

The suppressive effects of curcumin on macrophage migration were further demonstrated in another mouse study. In that study, adipose (fatty) tissue was taken from mice fed a high fat diet and then cultured to create an adipose-tissue solution. This solution was then introduced to a cell line of macrophages. When it was, the pro-inflammatory properties of the marcophages were activated, along with a release of MCP-1. But once curcumin was added to the solution, the macrophages' pro-inflammatory responses were reduced, as were the levels of MCP-1. Based on these findings, the researchers wrote that curcumin can restrain "obesity-induced inflammatory responses by suppressing adipose tissue macrophage accumulation or activation and inhibiting MCP-1," and thus has the potential to "improve chronic inflammatory conditions in obesity."

Human studies have also demonstrated the ability of turmeric and curcumin to reduce chronic inflammation. Earlier in this chapter you learned that one of the primary markers for, and indicators of, chronic inflammation is C-reactive protein, or CRP. Research has clearly demonstrated that curcumin and other curcuminoids that turmeric contains can significantly reduce CRP levels in as little as four weeks. Among such studies confirming this fact is a meta-analysis that was published in the science journal *Phytotherapy Research*.

The meta-analysis examined the results of six clinical trials conducted on a total of 172 subjects who received curcuminoids and 170 other subjects who received placebos. The studies were carried out over different durations, ranging from six days to three months. Overall, the test subjects who received the curcuminoids had CRP levels that were lower than the placebo test subjects by an average of 6.55 milligrams per liter (mg/L). The results were most significant in the studies that ran for at least four weeks. As I wrote above, any reading that is less than 10 mg/L is considered a normal CRP level. But an optimal range for CRP is less than 1.0 mg/L in women and below 0.55 mg/L in men.

As the author of the meta-analysis noted, the mechanisms of action involved in the ability of the cucurminoids found in turmeric to lower CRP include the suppression of the NF-kappaB pathway that results in the production of pro-inflammatory cytokines, as well as the ability of these turmeric compounds to reduce the release of pro-inflammatory cytokines via other signaling pathways. Based on the findings of the meta-analysis, Dr. Amirhossein Sahebkar, who conducted it, suggested that curcuminoids could be used in conjunction with statin drugs to lower the CRP levels of patients with cardiovascular disease (CVD) to achieve "a significantly greater reduction in CRP levels and incidence of primary and secondary CVD events."

The above studies are only a few of many others that also have found how and why turmeric and curcumin provide potent anti-inflammatory benefits. Throughout the rest of this book, you will learn of other such studies and the benefits that both turmeric and curcumin provide for specific diseases known to be caused by chronic inflammation.

CONCLUSION

By now you should have a clearer understanding of why chronic inflammation poses such a danger to your health, and also why it acts as a primary causative factor in so many debilitating and degenerative diseases. Just as importantly, you now know why turmeric, along with its key ingredient, curcumin, can go a long way towards preventing chronic inflammation, as well as helping to reverse it when it is already present. And you also know which tests you can request from your doctor to determine whether or not you currently suffer from chronic inflammation.

In the following chapters, we are going to examine more closely how chronic inflammation acts to trigger specific diseases, and how turmeric can act as a powerful natural healing aid to both prevent and help reverse such conditions. We will start with a look at the important benefits turmeric can provide for your brain, including protecting it from Alzheimer's disease, dementia, and depression.

3

A New Hope for Alzheimer's Disease, Dementia & Other Brain Disorders

Some of the most significant health benefits turmeric and curcumin provide have to do with how they protect the brain. As you will learn in this chapter, this is particularly true with regard to Alzheimer's disease and dementia, as well as other brain-related conditions, such as depression. First, let's begin by taking a closer look at the brain itself.

Your brain is what makes you human. It has shaped your personality, provided you with the capacity to read and understand these words and master your language, and given you the capacity to think, decide, distinguish right from wrong, create, and interact and successfully cope with the outside world. Your brain also controls every function in your body, from your ability to breathe and move, to orchestrating and overseeing all of the untold, moment-to-moment processes carried out by your body's trillions of cells. Without your brain, you could not process and make sense of the constant stream of sensory data that bombards your senses each and every moment of your life, including when you are sleeping, nor could you remember and learn from your past experiences and memories, every single one of them having been recorded by your brain's neurons.

Yet, today your brain is under more assaults than ever before, which is why in recent decades, there has been a frightening surge in the incidence of brain diseases such as Alzheimer's and dementia. As with many other degenerative diseases, such types of brain disease were once rare. Now, they are not only becoming commonplace, they are manifesting earlier than ever before. Where only a few short decades ago, conditions such as Alzheimer's and dementia seemed to manifest only in old age, today they are afflicting otherwise seemingly healthy men and women in their 50s and, in some cases, even earlier.

Consider these facts:

- One in eight Americans sixty-five or older has Alzheimer's disease.

- Forty-five percent of all Americans eighty-five or older have Alzheimer's.

- Nearly five percent of all Americans below the age of sixty-five are also afflicted with Alzheimer's.

- Alzheimer's disease is the sixth leading cause of death in the United States.

The statistics on dementia among Americans is equally grim, with incidences projected to double every twenty years. *Dementia* is an umbrella term used to describe a variety of diseases and conditions that develop when nerve cells in the brain die or no longer function normally. The death or malfunction of these nerve cells, called neurons, causes changes in one's memory, behavior, and ability to think clearly. These changes eventually impair the brain's ability to properly oversee such basic bodily functions as walking and swallowing.

It is commonly assumed that the rise in Alzheimer's and dementia rates are primarily due to the fact that, overall, Americans are living longer than their ancestors. That assumption is erroneous. There are far more important factors involved that can take hold many years, and even decades, prior to symptoms of such conditions first becoming noticeable. Recognizing and addressing those factors before they become severe is the key to keeping your brain healthy and youthful.

Fortunately, your brain is one of the most adaptable and resilient organs in your body. When provided with what it needs to be healthy, it can exhibit remarkable powers of regeneration and renewal.

HOW INFLAMMATION HARMS YOUR BRAIN

Research has demonstrated that chronic inflammation anywhere in your body can have a negative effect on the health of your brain and how it functions. Additionally, scientists have also discovered that another significant cause of impaired brain function is brain inflammation, also known as *neuro-inflammation*. Just as chronic inflammation in the rest of your body can cause a wide range of health problems, it can also trigger brain and cognitive problems. In fact, inflammation in the brain and elsewhere in the body creates a vicious cycle.

As you learned earlier in this book, whenever inflammation occurs in the body it causes the release of cytokines, especially within the immune system.

Scientists have discovered that these cytokines are capable of transmitting messages across the blood-brain barrier that can trigger inflammation in the brain. Left unchecked, this process has been found to negatively impact brain function and destroy brain tissue. As it occurs, inflammation in the brain can also initiate or further exacerbate chronic inflammation elsewhere in the body, causing joint pain, pain in the gastrointestinal tract, and other symptoms.

A growing body of research is establishing the link between impaired brain health, chronic inflammation, and autoimmune responses in which the body's immune system attacks healthy tissues and organs. Studies have also linked brain inflammation to chronic depression. When inflammation in the brain occurs, the rate at which neurons fire slows down. This, in turn, can lead to brain fog and impaired memory. Brain inflammation also reduces energy production in brain cells. Chronic brain inflammation can lead to neuron death and the onset of neurodegenerative diseases.

The primary cells of the brain that are affected by inflammation are called *microglia,* which act as the first and main type of active immune defense in the brain and central nervous system. Under healthy conditions, microglia perform and maintain numerous important functions that help ensure healthy function and protect the brain from inflammation and premature aging. But when they interact with toxins, bacteria, or other foreign matter that penetrate into the brain due to a leaky blood-brain barrier, they trigger an inflammatory immune response.

Because microglia have no "off switch," once they become activated, they will continue to promote brain inflammation for the rest of their lifespan, causing the destruction of brain tissue and increasing the risk of brain degeneration. Additionally, once activated, microglia typically activate other surrounding microglia, creating a domino effect of ever-worsening inflammation in the brain.

Based on these facts, you can see why inflammation poses such a serious threat to the health of your brain, as well as to your overall health.

OTHER RISK FACTORS
THAT CAN DAMAGE YOUR BRAIN

A variety of other factors can also harm your brain, and also act as additional triggers of neuro-inflammation. When faced with these persistent risk factors, your brain can become overburdened, and eventually, if they are not properly dealt with and reversed, impaired brain function will result.

What follows is an overview of some of the most common other risk factors that can negatively affect brain health.

Fascinating Facts About Your Brain

The adult human brain weighs approximately three pounds (1.4 kilograms), which is no more than 2 percent of the total body weight for most adult men. In appearance, it resembles a mass of jelly. In order to function properly, your brain requires lots of oxygen and energy. It uses 20 percent of your body's total daily energy and oxygen supply.

On average, brains in adult males are approximately 10 percent larger than female brains, even after the larger body size of males compared to females is taken into account. The larger brain size in men is not an indication of superior brain function, however. If brain size correlated to superior function, then our Neanderthal ancestors would have been better equipped than we are to face the modern world, since their brains were 10 percent larger than ours are. In fact, our brains are continuing to become smaller, with scientists estimating that human brain size has shrunk by the size of a tennis ball over the past 10 to 20,000 years.

Although most people think their brains are solid, in reality, like the rest of the human body, the brain is mostly composed of water, which comprises approximately 73 percent of its mass. For this reason, chronic low-grade dehydration can impair healthy brain function, affecting memory and other cognitive skills.

The rest of your brain is comprised mostly of fats and proteins, with 60 percent of its solid mass made up of fats, making your brain the fattiest organ is your body. Healthy brain function depends on a regular supply of healthy fats, including saturated fats, in your diet.

One quarter (25 percent) of the cholesterol produced by your body

Poor Diet and Nutritional Deficiencies

Poor diet and nutritional deficiencies are a primary cause of brain degeneration. Deficiencies in various vitamins, minerals, essential fatty acids, and amino acids, including those found in turmeric, have all been linked to impaired brain function, as well as brain diseases, including Alzheimer's and dementia. These deficiencies are compounded by unhealthy diets, which not only prevent your brain from getting all of the nutrients it needs, but also results in over-acidity, chronic inflammation, and blood sugar imbalances.

One of the main reasons why a healthy diet and a daily supply of nutrients are so essential for proper brain function has to with how the brain operates. It does so primarily through the transmission of chemical messengers known ends up in the brain, because cholesterol is an essential component of every brain cell. Without enough cholesterol, brain cells will die. High total cholesterol levels have also been shown to reduce the risk of dementia and Alzheimer's disease.

There are an estimated 86 billion cells in the human brain, but not all brain cells are alike. In addition, there are approximately 10,000 different types of neurons in the brain. Each neuron connects with an average of 40,000 synapses, with all neurons and synapses communicating with each other.

The human brain does not fully mature until around twenty-five years of age. Until recently, it was thought that once full brain maturity was achieved, the brain's neural pathways were set for the rest of one's life, and no new neural pathways were capable of being formed. Scientists now know this is not true. New neural pathways can be formed at any age so long as the brain remains healthy. The brain's ongoing ability to form new neural pathways is known as *neuroplasticity.*

Your brain generates electricity, producing an average of twelve to twenty-five watts of electricity per day, which is enough energy to power a low-watt LED light bulb. Over 100,000 chemical reactions occur within your brain every second.

Within your brain, there are approximately 400 miles of blood vessels. Contrary to popular opinion, we do not use only 10 percent of our brains. Brain scans reveal that we use almost all parts of our brains all of the time, including when we are sleeping.

Although your experience of pain is processed by the brain, the brain itself is incapable of feeling pain because it has no pain receptors, unlike all other organs in your body.

as *neurotransmitters,* which are responsible for how the brain communicates with the rest of the body. For neurotransmitters to be able to transmit the brain's messages effectively, an adequate supply of brain nutrients is necessary. When the supply of nutrients is insufficient, the brain and its functions are adversely affected.

Environmental Toxins

It is well known that environmental toxins play a significant role in various neurological conditions, in addition to other degenerative diseases, such as cancer, diabetes, and heart disease. Environmental toxins harm the brain both directly, by crossing the blood-brain barrier, and indirectly, by compromising immune and liver function. This includes fluoride, which is found in much of our nation's water supply despite being a known neurotoxin.

Toxins that cross the blood-brain barrier deposit themselves within brain tissues, causing brain cells, tissues, and neurotransmitters to become impaired, and eventually leading to the buildup of brain plaque, which is a major contributing factor in the onset of Alzheimer's and dementia. This process is further exacerbated by the negative effects toxins have on the immune system and the liver.

Altered immune function caused by environmental toxins causes the blood-brain barrier to become more porous, or "leaky," in much the same way that toxins can cause leaky gut syndrome. The more porous the blood-brain barrier becomes, the easier it is for toxins to cross it and settle in brain tissue.

Blood Sugar Imbalances

Stable blood sugar (glucose) levels are essential for healthy brain function. Blood sugar levels that are too high (hyperglycemia), too low (hypoglycemia), or which regularly fluctuate between levels that are high and low, can all impair your brain's ability to perform its many tasks.

The reason blood sugar levels are such vital factors in brain health is because glucose is the brain's primary source of fuel. Optimal blood sugar levels help ensure that overall brain chemistry remains balanced, and also prevent damage to, or loss of, neuron structure and function, as well as the death of neurons. Balanced blood sugar levels are also required for the proper production of neurotransmitters, as well as healthy neurotransmitter metabolism and function.

Unbalanced, or unstable, blood sugar levels either deprive the brain of enough glucose or flood it with too much glucose. Either way, brain health is negatively impacted. Brain symptoms caused or made worse by low blood sugar include excess production of the adrenal hormones epinephrine and norepinephrine, as a result of low levels of the adrenal hormone cortisol. Cortisol, as mentioned earlier, prevents low blood sugar. Other symptoms caused by low blood sugar include mood swings, anxiety, irritability, forgetfulness, and feelings of lightheadedness.

High blood sugar levels result in insulin resistance, as the pancreas continues to produce insulin in an effort to force glucose into the cells. However, the excess glucose gets converted into fat, increasing total body fat. The conversion of glucose into fat requires energy, which creates adrenal fatigue. High insulin levels cause chronic inflammation, disruption of other hormones, and impaired neurotransmitter function, all of which, in turn, can cause degeneration of the brain and its functions. In addition, elevated blood sugar and insulin resistance also cause excessive production of cortisol.

Oxygen Supply

A sufficient supply of oxygen to the brain is one of the most important requirements for healthy brain function. In fact, oxygen deprivation lasting more than five minutes is all that is usually necessary to cause permanent brain damage. Signs of a lack of brain oxygen include poor focus and concentration, cold extremities (hands and feet), poor finger- and toenail health, and fungal growth on the toes.

Most of us typically believe we are getting all of the oxygen we need simply because we are still breathing. However, most people are habitually shallow breathers and are thus deprived of an adequate supply of oxygen on a daily basis.

Oxygen is carried to your brain by your blood, which also transports the nutrients, hormones, and neurotransmitters that your brain requires. Poor blood flow, or circulation, is the primary cause of lack of oxygen in the brain, and also the cause of vascular dementia, which is the second most common form of dementia after Alzheimer's disease. Lack of oxygen also prevents brain neurons from producing all of the energy they need to survive and carry out their many functions. In short, poor circulation and lack of oxygen to the brain go hand in hand.

Hormone Imbalances

Healthy hormone function is also essential for a healthy, optimally functioning brain. Both brain neurons and various brain cells have receptor sites for hormones, and research has shown that healthy hormone balance plays important roles in preventing brain inflammation and degeneration, as well as in helping neural networks to grow and branch out, and in maintaining optimal neuroplasticity. Hormones also help to maintain the shape and structure of the brain. Hormone imbalances can seriously impair all the above functions, as well as accelerate premature aging of the brain.

Pharmaceutical Drugs

The ongoing use of pharmaceutical drugs is one of the primary causes of dementia and other brain conditions, including delirium, in the elderly. This is especially true of people who have been prescribed more than one drug at a time. This is known as drug-induced cognitive impairment.

Given how widespread the use of pharmaceutical drugs has become in our society, drug-induced brain problems no longer affect just the elderly.

This is not surprising, since all pharmaceutical drugs carry some risk of side effects. Common side effects related to the brain that can be caused by regular drug use also include anxiety, "brain fog," depression, erratic behavior patterns, and suicidal thoughts. In certain cases, drugs, either alone or used in combination, can even cause brain damage.

Many drugs can also interfere with the brain's ability to produce energy because of how they impair mitochondria function. Mitochondria act as your cells' energy plants. Among the highest concentrations of mitochondria in the body are those within the brain and the heart.

Another area of concern regarding brain health is the potentially harmful role that statin drugs may play. Statins, which act to lower cholesterol levels in the body, represent the most widely prescribed class of drugs in the United States today. Although many physicians still believe otherwise, a growing body of research has clearly demonstrated that cholesterol, in and of itself, is not a risk factor for heart disease. It only becomes so when it is oxidized, which is what happens when the body is subjected to chronic inflammation. (For more on this, see Chapter 5.) Cholesterol plays many important roles in helping the body to maintain its health, including within the brain and nervous system.

One of the most important roles cholesterol plays is in the formation of synapses, or connections between neurons. Synapse formation is directly dependent on cholesterol, and without enough of it, proper learning and memory function cannot take place. In fact, one of the reasons that healthy sleep is beneficial to learning and memory is because it enables the brain to make more cholesterol. Because of how statins inhibit cholesterol levels, a number of health experts speculate that the rising rates of Alzheimer's and dementia over the past few decades may, at least indirectly, be related to the corresponding increase in statin use over that same time period.

(If you are currently using prescription drugs and suspect they may be affecting your brain function, speak with your doctor. In almost all cases, normal brain function can be reversed or returned to its pre-drug state by stopping the use of the offending drug. The weaning off process needs to be supervised by a physician.)

Lack of Sleep

As it is for the rest of your body, sleep is the time of repair for your brain. During sleep, your brain also consolidates the memories of what you learned and experienced during the day. Sleep also aids your brain in ridding itself of wastes.

Numerous previous studies have demonstrated how important healthy sleep is for brain health, and how fitful sleep can negatively impact the brain and its many functions. Lack of sleep has also been found to be a contributing factor in the development of Alzheimer's and dementia. Therefore, ensuring that you obtain adequate amounts of quality sleep each night is vitally important for maintaining the optimal brain health.

Fast Facts About Alzheimer's Disease

Alzheimer's disease was named after the German psychologist and neuropathologist Alois Alzheimer (1865–1915), who discovered it in 1906. It was once a rare condition, but has become increasingly prevalent in recent decades, both in the United States and in many other countries around the world, especially in those who follow diets similar to the nutritionally deficient standard American diet.

The following are some important facts about Alzheimer's disease:

- Today, over five million Americans suffer from Alzheimer's disease, and it is estimated that this number will more than triple over the next few decades.

- Alzheimer's is the most prevalent form of dementia, accounting for an estimated 70 percent of all cases of dementia in the United States.

- At present, Alzheimer's disease is the sixth leading cause of death in the United States.

- According to the Alzheimer's Association, a research organization, every sixty-six seconds one more person develops Alzheimer's in the United States. That equates to more than 1,300 new cases every single day.

- For reasons that scientists have yet to fully understand, women are twice as likely as men to develop Alzheimer's, according to data compiled by the United States Department of Health and Human Services (HHS).

- Contrary to popular belief, Alzheimer's disease does not always begin in old age, but can actually begin to develop as early as one's thirties and forties, going undiagnosed and unsuspected for decades before its first tangible symptoms become evident.

- By 2050, the Alzheimer's Association projects that the medical cost of treating Alzheimer's disease in the United States alone will exceed one trillion dollars each year.

TURMERIC AND CURCUMIN FOR BRAIN HEALTH

An ongoing body of research continues to establish the fact that both turmeric and curcumin can play important roles in protecting the brain and keeping it healthy throughout one's life. They are able to do so primarily because of the anti-inflammatory benefits that they provide. Their proven ability to act as natural antioxidants is vital in this regard, as well. Perhaps even more important, however, is the fact that turmeric, and especially curcumin, are both capable of crossing the blood-brain barrier to directly access the brain itself and provide a variety of neuroprotective benefits.

Curcumin's brain-enhancing benefits in particular are most remarkable. This fact was demonstrated by a study published in the *Journal of Psychopharmacology,* which showed that a single dose (400 mg) of a curcumin supplement was capable of boosting memory within one hour after it was administered. In the study, which involved sixty healthy adults between the ages of sixty to eighty-five, participants underwent a variety of tests, including memory assessment and attention tasks, both before and one hour after they received the curcumin supplement. Compared to a placebo group, the curcumin group exhibited significantly improved memory and attention performance only one hour after taking the supplement. This was also true when the participants were again tested three hours after taking curcumin.

The study participants continued to receive the same dose of curcumin as a supplement for an additional four weeks, after which time they were once again tested to assess their memory and other cognitive skills. According to the researchers, "Working memory and mood (general fatigue and change in state calmness, contentedness and fatigue induced by psychological stress) were significantly better following chronic [daily] treatment. A significant acute-on-chronic treatment effect on alertness and contentedness was also observed."

In addition, the researchers also discovered that daily supplementation with curcumin "was associated with significantly reduced total and LDL cholesterol" levels. While, as I mentioned, cholesterol itself is not a danger to your health, this finding is still worth noting since scientists now know that there is a direct correlation between brain and heart health.

It is studies like the one above that have led to ongoing research into the potential benefits turmeric and curcumin may hold for these diseases. Scientists have observed that people who regularly consume curries and other foods in which turmeric is an ingredient typically exhibit a lower incidence of Alzheimer's disease and dementia as they age, compared to their counterparts here in the United States and other Western nations. These observations have spurred interest in further research into this area.

A Curious Finding

The potential that a turmeric-rich diet has for lowering the incidence of Alzheimer's disease and dementia is all the more intriguing when we consider the fact that in India, where curries are a staple food, the percentage of people between the ages of seventy to seventy-nine who are affected by these conditions is less than 25 percent of the rate in the United States for people in the same age group. The incidence of Alzheimer's among this same age group in the United States is 4.4 times higher than that of its Indian counterparts.

Intrigued by this fact, researchers obtained permission to conduct autopsies of the brains of men and women in India who had died from all causes. What they found surprised them. The tissues of the brains, particularly tissues in the region of the hippocampus, the brain's primary "memory center," were found to be colored with the same yellowish hue of turmeric. When similar brain autopsies were performed on people from other nations, no such coloring was found, leading the researchers to conclude that not only does turmeric cross the blood-brain barrier, but when it does so, it is readily absorbed by brain tissues, where it acts protectively.

A Look at Alzheimer's and Dementia

Alzheimer's and dementia in general are particularly insidious diseases because of how they slowly, yet steadily, develop, often over decades, before their symptoms at last become apparent and are properly diagnosed. By then, for the vast majority of people who suffer from these conditions, such symptoms are considered irreversible, at least according to conventional medicine. That's because, despite the tens of billions of dollars that have been spent worldwide since the start of the twenty-first century to develop a drug capable of slowing the development of Alzheimer's and dementia, all the drugs that have been developed thus far have been abject failures. And that's just in respect to *slowing* these conditions, not actually stopping and reversing their progression.

Given such poor outcomes, some researchers today are even questioning the wisdom of continuing to fund research to find a drug-based solution for Alzheimer's. Instead, they are recommending shifting research funds to investigate the potential of diet and nutrition to both prevent and help reverse Alzheimer's and dementia. In line with their recommendations, a portion of research funding for these conditions has shifted into this area, with turmeric, and especially curcumin, being two of the most widely studied nutritional approaches that are being investigated. Thus far, research has demonstrated that both substances hold great promise for Alzheimer's and dementia patients.

To better understand why, first let's take a look at the factors that are involved in the onset and progression of Alzheimer's disease and dementia. (Since the terms *Alzheimer's disease* and *dementia* are often used interchangeably, and the conditions themselves are for the most part indistinguishable, I will use *Alzheimer's* alone from this point forward.)

Currently, scientists know that Alzheimer's develops as a result of changes in the brain's neurons, particularly those located in the hippocampus region, which oversees memory functions. Neurons, which are also know as nerve fibers, receive, process, and transmit information from the brain to the rest of the body via their chemical and electrical activity within the body's nervous system. In the case of Alzheimer's, neurons can become damaged or impaired by the buildup of substances called *beta-amyloid plaques.* These plaques are composed of proteins, and under normal circumstances they are eliminated from the brain after they have performed their intended functions. In Alzheimer's, however, instead of being eliminated, they accumulate, causing the plaques they form to grow as well, harming the brain's neuronal system.

Another class of proteins, known as *tau proteins,* or tau fibers, is also involved in the development and progression of Alzheimer's. Tau proteins are found in abundance within neurons, and are necessary for stabilizing what are known as *microtubules.* Microtubules are long, hollow cylinders that play many important roles in the cells, including brain cells, and also help to maintain cell structure. Tau proteins, in turn, help to stabilize microtubules. In cases of Alzheimer's, tau proteins become tangled within neurons, further damaging neuronal functions, including memory.

In addition to the buildup of beta-amyloid plaques and the formation of tangled tau proteins, scientists also know that both chronic inflammation and oxidative stress (see Chapter 2) are also involved in the onset of Alzheimer's. In fact, recent research has shown that the pro-inflammatory and oxidative processes that play primary roles in the development of type 2, or adult-onset diabetes, are very similar to how inflammation and oxidative stress affect the brain. For this reason, some researchers now refer to Alzheimer's as "type 3 diabetes."

Knowing the above facts, let's now return to examining how and why turmeric and curcumin are showing great promise in preventing and treating Alzheimer's.

The first reason, as you learned in Chapter 2, is because of how both turmeric and curcumin are able to successfully prevent and reverse chronic inflammation. And, because of the abilities of both turmeric and curcumin to cross the blood-brain barrier, they are able to prevent and reverse inflammation within the brain itself, not just in the body. This is vitally important and something that few other nutrients are capable of doing. Nor can any of the drugs that are currently being used by physicians to treat Alzheimer's, which helps to explain why the effectiveness of such drugs is so poor.

The anti-inflammatory benefits that both turmeric and curcumin have for protecting the health of the brain are also matched by both substances' proven antioxidant benefits. Both animal and human studies have demonstrated that curcumin, for example, once it penetrates into the brain, is capable of minimizing and protecting against free damage in brain cells and tissues because of it antioxidant, free radical-quenching properties. In a study of mice with induced Alzheimer's symptoms, curcumin was shown to reduce the oxidation of the proteins that make up beta-amyloid. This has been borne out by human studies, as well. These findings are important because the oxidation of such proteins is a primary factor involved in the creation and accumulation of beta-amyloid plaques in the brain.

Of equal importance are animal and human studies which show that curcumin also helps protect against free radical damage to the brain's neurovascular system. By doing so, curcumin helps to maintain the blood-brain barrier so that it can more effectively prevent toxins and other harmful substances from entering and taking hold in brain cells and tissues. Moreover, curcumin's protective benefits for the neurovascular system have also been found to help prevent and reduce the effects of vascular dementia.

In addition, research on both curcumin and turmeric has been shown to prevent brain cell damage and death by inhibiting pro-inflammatory, oxidizing cells known as cytokines, as well as COX-2 enzymes. Cytokines and COX-2 enzymes are both involved in the body's natural processes of inflammation that protect against infectious microorganisms and help speed the healing of wounds and other injuries. But they also play major roles in triggering and exacerbating chronic inflammation in both the body and the brain, and can act as co-factors in the onset of Alzheimer's.

Besides taming inflammation and free radical damage in the brain, turmeric and, most especially, curcumin also provide direct benefits as natural treatments for beta-amyloid plaques and tangled tau proteins. This has been confirmed in *in vitro* (lab tests in which curcumin or turmeric was introduced to isolated brain cell lines and tissues, as well as beta-amyloid plaques) animal and human studies.

Based on the results of these studies, researchers have concluded that turmeric and curcumin clear beta-amyloid plaques from the brain by binding to and dissolving them, causing them to be excreted into the bloodstream for elimination from the body. They also inhibit the plaques' production by first inhibiting the growth of beta-amyloid itself, as well as other substances that contribute to their development. Finally, they reduce toxicity in the brain caused by the plaques. It was also concluded that turmeric and curcumin rid the brain of tangled tau proteins in the same way they do beta-amyloid plaques, as well as hinder their production and progression.

In addition to the recently referenced mechanisms, studies have also shown that turmeric and curcumin help to prevent cholesterol in the brain from becoming oxidized. Oxidized cholesterol, especially LDL cholesterol, is not only a major risk factor for heart disease and stroke, but has also been implicated as a factor involved in the onset of Alzheimer's and dementia. Researchers have also found that turmeric and curcumin act as natural chelating agents that help to remove heavy metals from brain cells and tissues, especially excess iron and fluoride. Accumulations of both these and other metals have long been associated with an increased risk for Alzheimer's and other brain disorders.

A Study on Curcumin for Dementia

One of the most remarkable studies that reveals the potential that turmeric holds for Alzheimer's was conducted by Japanese researchers and published in the Indian medical journal *Ayu*. It involved three patients (two females and one male). Describing them, the researchers wrote, "Their cognitive decline and Behavioral and Psychological Symptoms of Dementia (BPSD) were very severe. All three patients exhibited irritability, agitation, anxiety, and apathy, two patients suffer from urinary incontinence and wanderings." All of the above symptoms are commonly experienced by people who suffer from Alzheimer's and dementia, and typically worsen as these diseases progress.

Each of the study participants were given a daily dose of turmeric powder (764 mg of turmeric with a standardized amount of 100 mg/day of curcumin). Within twelve weeks, all of them began "recovering from these symptoms without any adverse reaction in the clinical symptom and laboratory data," and within that same period the researchers reported, the patients' "total score of the Neuro Psychiatric Inventory-brief Questionnaire decreased significantly in both acuity [severity] of symptoms and burden of caregivers."

In their published study, the researchers provided case studies of each of the study participants. What follow are excerpts from each of them.

Case One

The focus of the first case was an eighty-year-old female with progressive dementia who "had started to exhibit disturbances of short-term memory and orientation when she was seventy-six years old. . . . She also had difficulty in learning new information. Gradually, her daily activity was disturbed. [The woman] had increasing difficulty in getting dressed, cooking, and coordination household tasks.

"She wandered aimlessly around the house, had incontinence of urine, [and] some psychobehavioral changes, such as apathy, anxiety, agitation, and irritability. She required the presence of a caregiver, though she was prescribed AChEl inhibitor (donepezil 10 mg) and *Yokukansan,* which is a traditional Japanese medicine (Kampo).

"When she was eighty-three years old, she scored on 1/30 her Mini-Mental State Examination (MMSE), which was used for evaluation of cognitive functions. . . . After turmeric 764 mg/day (curcumin 100 mg/day) treatment for twelve weeks, both scores of acuity of symptoms and burden of caregivers were decreased by the Japanese version of Neuropsychiatric Inventory-brief Questionnaire (NPI-Q) Among the NPI-Q subscales, her agitation, apathy, anxiety, and irritability were relieved."

The researchers added that the woman also began to inform her caregivers when she needed to urinate, and started to enjoy and share in the laughter of others as they watched comedy programs on TV. She also started to sing songs and to knit, both of which were activities she used to do before her illness. Most importantly, within one year of supplementing with turmeric, the woman once again came to recognize her family members. The researchers concluded by writing that "she lives a peaceful life without significant BPSD."

Case Two

The symptoms of an eighty-four-year-old female with progressive Alzheimer's included "forgetfulness, disorientation to place and time, hallucination, delusion, agitation, irritability, depression, apathy, confabulation [false memories], wandering, and incontinence of urine, which developed several years prior. . . . At the time of her initial visit, her cognitive decline was already very severe and her MMSE score was 0/30 . . . cerebral MRI revealed moderate bilateral temporal atrophy with the mild ventricular dilation.

"AChEl inhibitor (donepezil) could not [be used] because of the side effects. The woman's BPSD, including agitation, irritability, and anxiety, was not improved, though she was prescribed *Yokukansan* and atypical antipsychotic drugs. We began to administer turmeric 764 mg/day (curcumin 100 mg/day) to her.

"She gradually calmed down. Her BPSD, which were hallucination, delusion, depression, agitation, apathy, anxiety, and irritability, were relieved. She stopped urinating outside the front door. She came to put on her clothes properly, and distinguish her family from staff of the care center. After twelve weeks, judging from the Japanese version of NPI-Q, both acuity of BPSD and burden of caregivers were relieved. . . . She has been taking turmeric for more than one year. She lives in a peacefully serene manner with her family."

Case Three

The third case began, "A seventy-nine-year-old male patient presented [himself] at our hospital, accompanied by his wife. She reported that the short-term memory loss gradually developed over several years, though he was already prescribed AChEl inhibitor (donepezil 5 mg) by his previous doctor for three years. He wanted to stay at home, and lived an idle life. He stopped painting in oils, which he used to do for his hobby. . . .

"Routine blood tests were normal, including thyroid function, serum vitamin B_1, B_{12}, and folic acid. Cerebral MRI demonstrated mild bilateral temporal atrophy with mild ischemic changes in deep white matter. Single-Photon Emission Computed Tomography showed typical AD [Alzheimer's disease] pattern . . . His MMSE score was 12/30, with poor orientation to place and time, calculation, concentration, recall . . . spontaneous writing, and verbal fluency.

His BPSD were agitation, depression, apathy, anxiety, euphoria, aberrant eating behavior, and irritability. Turmeric 764 mg/day (curcumin 100 mg/day) treatment for twelve weeks relieved the patient's BPSD, especially agitation, irritability, and depression. Both scores of acuity of symptoms and burden of the caregivers were decreased. . . . His MMSE score was up five points, [at] 17/30. . . . He has been taking turmeric for more than one year. He lives calmly with his wife."

A Doctor's Approach to Treating Alzheimer's with Curcumin

One of the foremost experts and researchers in the field of Alzheimer's disease and dementia is Dale E. Bredeson, MD, founding president and CEO of the Buck Institute for Research on Aging in Novato, California, and author of the book *The End of Alzheimer's*. Recognizing the severe limitations and side effects of current medications used to treat patients with Alzheimer's and dementia, Dr. Bredeson has developed a comprehensive nutritional and lifestyle program, which has been medically proven to not only slow the progression of these diseases, but to actually begin to reverse and possibly cure them. His research and work with Alzheimer's and dementia patients has garnered him international acclaim because of the results he is achieving.

Curcumin is among the nutritional supplements Dr. Bredeson uses as part of his overall Alzheimer's treatment program, which is known as ReCode. He employs it specifically to reduce C-reactive protein (CRP), a marker for inflammation associated with Alzheimer's, and to reduce levels of beta amyloid in the brain. Given the fact that one of the world's top experts in the treating of Alzheimer's is using curcumin as part of his overall protocol, doesn't it make good sense that you should consider using it, too?

TWO WAYS CURCUMIN MIGHT HELP PREVENT/TREAT ALZHEIMER'S DISEASE AND DEMENTIA

Researchers continue to discover the potential that turmeric and curcumin hold as safe, effective, and inexpensive aids for preventing and dealing with Alzheimer's disease and dementia. As they do so, they have uncovered two additional ways that these natural substances can further help ward off these conditions, as well as the potential they hold for helping physicians identify and diagnose Alzheimer's, including in its earliest stages.

Creating New Neurons

It was only in recent decades that scientists discovered that the human brain and its brain cells and network of neurons have the capacity to continue to grow. Previously, it was considered a scientific fact that, once the brain grew to adult size, no additional brain cells, including neurons, could be grown. In other words, scientists believed the brain you had by your early twenties was in its peak state of development, after which time it would begin to age and decline as brain cells began to die off, never to be replaced. Scientists now know this isn't true. Your brain can and does continue to grow as you go through life, and it is capable of growing new brain cells. This process is known as *neurogenesis.*

According to a scientific overview of the benefits that curcumin provides for Alzheimer's that was published in the prestigious *British Medical Journal,* a number of research studies have demonstrated that it can and does stimulate new brain cell growth, including the growth of new neurons. Since neurons are damaged or destroyed as Alzheimer's develops, curcumin's ability to stimulate neurogenesis is highly significant. Of even more significance is the fact that researchers have found that curcumin helps to stimulate the growth of new neurons in the hippocampus region of the brain, the "seat of memory" that is most affected by Alzheimer's. Researchers have also found that a turmeric-rich diet can provide similar benefits.

Curcumin and Epigenetics

Just as scientists once believed that the human brain did not continue to develop and grow new brain cells, so they also formerly believed that the genes we are born with meant that our "genetic destiny" was set in stone and could not be altered. We now know that this isn't true, either.

While it is certainly true that our genes, specifically our DNA, do predispose us to certain experiences in life, including certain disease conditions, scientists now know that it is not so much the genes themselves that matter, but whether or not they become triggered, or activated. A wide variety of factors, both external (such as poor diet and environmental triggers, including toxins) and internal (such as chronic stress), play key roles in whether or not genes associated with specific diseases become activated or remain dormant. The study of these factors is known as *epigenetics.*

While a growing body of research continues to find that certain genes or gene clusters do, in fact, serve as indicators of a genetic *predisposition* for developing certain conditions, studies have also now revealed that, in order for you to actually develop those conditions, the associated predisposing genes need to first be activated. This activation process is known as *gene expression.* Epigenetic researchers investigate the conditions that trigger gene expression.

Scientists now know that epigenetic factors also play important roles in determining whether or not a person will develop Alzheimer's. They have also found that a specific gene known as ApoE4 (apolipoprotein E4) indicates a predisposition for Alzheimer's. However, carriers of the ApoE4 gene do not always develop the disease. Many do not and will not. Conversely, many people who lack the ApoE4 gene do or will develop Alzheimer's disease.

One of the primary epigenetic factors that scientists now know plays a significant role in the onset and progression of Alzheimer's is called *histone modification.* Histones are a class of protein clusters or "spools" around which DNA threads coil themselves. They are also involved in normal cell division, but when this process of cell division goes awry through histone modification, serious health problems can occur, including Alzheimer's. Research has now established that one of the other important ways that curcumin can help prevent the onset, and minimize the progression of, Alzheimer's disease is its ability to prevent histone modification. By doing so, curcumin has been shown to be able to have a positive, neutralizing effect on an otherwise major epigenetic trigger of Alzheimer's.

Curcumin as a Diagnostic Aid

One of the most challenging aspects of Alzheimer's disease is the fact that it is typically difficult to diagnose until its symptoms have fully manifested and become severe. As with all other disease conditions, early detection of Alzheimer's might greatly increase the likelihood that its progression could be slowed or even reversed.

Recent research is demonstrating that curcumin has the potential to aid physicians in making a definitive diagnosis of Alzheimer's. Curcumin's ability in this regard has to do with two of its properties. First, as you learned above, it is able to cross the blood-brain barrier and bind to the beta-amyloid plaques and tangled tau proteins that are known to play a major role in the development and progression of Alzheimer's. Additionally, curcumin has the ability to fluoresce, meaning that it emits light, giving it a fluorescent quality. As curcumin binds with beta-amyloid plaques and tangled tau proteins, its presence within them, coupled with its fluorescent properties, makes it easier for these Alzheimer-related plaques and protein tangles to be detected via magnetic resonance imaging (MRI), and even via retinal scans. This latter diagnostic method using curcumin is significant because researchers have now found that signs of Alzheimer's can actually appear and be detected in the retina before they can be detected in the brain itself.

This ability of curcumin and the studies that demonstrate it were discussed in the same scientific overview in the *British Medical Journal* that I mentioned above. In it, the authors wrote, "Importantly, the pathology in the retina was detected before the stage at which pathology in the brain could be detected, indicating that curcumin may have potential as a pre-clinical AD [Alzheimer's disease] biomarker. The research also supports the previous observation that curcumin has the ability to cross the BBB [blood-brain barrier], which is essential for its therapeutic efficacy."

If future research continues to bear out these facts, one day soon physicians may use curcumin prior to conducting retinal scans or MRIs of the brain in order to screen their patients for Alzheimer's. Detecting the disease as early as possible allows the best chance of arresting its progression.

CURCUMIN AS A POTENTIAL AID FOR MAJOR DEPRESSIVE DISORDERS

The incidence of chronic depression in the United States, as well as in many other Western nations, continues to rise, to the point where it has now reached epidemic levels. Chronic depression is typically treated with antidepressant drugs, especially a class of drugs known as SSRIs (selective serotonin reuptake inhibitors). However, such drugs carry the risk of serious side-effects, including triggering the urge to commit suicide or harm others.

In recent years, researchers have presented a growing body of evidence that curcumin may not only improve the results achieved by SSRIs and other antidepressants when it is used in conjunction with such drugs, but that it may also provide its own noteworthy antidepressant benefits without the risk of any harmful side effects. Studies have already demonstrated that curcumin has a positive effect on a number of physiological responses that are now known to be associated with depression and other mood disorders. This is particularly true of curcumin's anti-inflammatory and antioxidant properties, as both inflammation and oxidative stress are now known to trigger and exacerbate chronic depression, as well as other mood disorders.

What follows is a summary of two such studies that demonstrate curcumin's potential antidepressant benefits.

The first study, which was published in the *Journal of Affective Disorders,* involved fifty-six patients, all of whom were diagnosed with major depressive disorder (MDD). As its name implies, MDD is a serious form of chronic depression. In the study, which was randomized, double-blind, and placebo-controlled, the patients were divided into two groups. The first group received a curcumin supplement as a capsule twice a day for a period of eight weeks. The second group received a placebo capsule during the same time period.

Prior to week four, both groups exhibited improvements in their MDD, but from the fourth week until the study's conclusion, those who were given curcumin capsules achieved significantly greater overall improvements compared to the placebo group. Moreover, these improvements were especially noteworthy in those whose cases of MDD were classified as atypical depression. Atypical depression is more difficult to treat than other types of MDD.

Prior to and after the eight-week study, researchers also collected blood, saliva, and urine samples from all of the study's participants in order to identify potential biomarkers associated with curcumin's anti-inflammatory effects in relation to MDD. Analysis of these samples found that curcumin improved levels of various anti-inflammatory markers. These findings further demonstrated curcumin's value as a natural antidepressant, since chronic inflammation is known to cause or exacerbate and prolong depression.

In another randomized, double-blind, placebo-controlled study that also involved patients with MDD, patients were again divided into two groups. The first group was treated with antidepressant drugs alone, while the second group received the same drugs, as well as curcumin supplements. By week six of the study, the curcumin group exhibited improvements in their MDD symptoms that were substantially greater than those who only received antidepressant drugs. Additionally, the curcumin group was also found to have decreased levels of inflammatory cytokines and the stress hormone cortisol, along with increased levels of specific proteins in the brain known as brain-derived neurotrophic factors (BDNFs) that are associated with non-depressive mental states. These BDNF proteins aid in the production and repair of brain cells and help to eliminate toxins in the brain. Based on this study's results, its authors wrote, "These findings indicate the potential benefits of . . . curcumin to reverse the development of depression and enhance the outcome of antidepressant treatments in major depressive disorder."

TURMERIC AND FLUORIDE

Despite being found in much of our nation's water supply, fluoride, even in small amounts, is a neurotoxin, meaning that it is capable of damaging the human brain and its functioning.

The addition of fluoride to the public water supply was initially done with the claim that fluoride reduces cavities and tooth decay. For this reason, fluoride is found in many commercial brands of toothpaste. However, this claim has been debunked by data compiled by the World Health Organization (WHO), which shows that there is little difference in the incidence of tooth decay and cavities between populations in municipalities with either fluoridated or non-fluoridated water supplies, and that, overall, the incidence of tooth decay has significantly declined at a similar rate in both populations.

Of far greater concern, however, is research showing that fluoride increases the risk of impaired fetal development and can result in lower IQ in children, and additional research that has found that fluoride causes calcification of the brain's pineal gland, which, among its other functions, is responsible for producing melatonin in the body and regulating the body's circadian rhythms and sleep cycle. In fact, the highest concentrations of fluoride in the body are found in the pineal gland. Other studies have linked fluoride to the development of various types of cancer, indicating that it is a carcinogen, as well as a mutagen, meaning that it is capable of altering and damaging cellular DNA.

For these and other reasons, the public water supplies of most developed nations around the world, including the vast majority of member nations of the European Union (EU), are fluoride-free. Major cities around the world that do not fluoridate their water include:

- Amsterdam
- Barcelona
- Basel
- Berlin
- Copenhagen
- Florence
- Frankfurt
- Geneva
- Glasgow

- Helsinki
- London
- Montreal
- Oslo

- Paris
- Rome
- Stockholm
- Tokyo

- Vancouver
- Venice
- Vienna
- Zurich

And since 2010, nearly 230 cities and townships in the United States and Canada have taken it upon themselves to remove fluoride from their water supplies, as well.

In addition to being found in many water supplies and in many brands of toothpaste and other dental products, fluoride is also contained in many commercial teas and tea drinks, as well as many sodas, commercial fruit and vegetable juices, and even beer. It is also commonly found in processed foods, contained in many pesticides, and is a component of many pharmaceutical drugs.

As with so many other toxins in our environment today, completely reducing your exposure to fluoride is virtually impossible. That is why it is so important to take measures that can protect you against fluoride and minimize its harmful effects. Turmeric and curcumin can both go a long way in helping you to do so, as animal studies have demonstrated.

In a study of mice, for example, researchers noted that curcumin "is known to have multiple activities, including an antioxidant property, and has been suggested to be useful in treatment of several neurological diseases." Therefore, they set out to investigate whether or not curcumin could minimize the effects of brain and neurotoxicity caused by having various groups of mice consume fluoridated water for thirty days. One group of mice consumed only fluoridated distilled water. A second group also consumed the same amount of fluoridated water to which a mixture of curcumin and olive oil (olive oil, along with other oils and foods containing fatty acids, improves the ability of curcumin to be absorbed by the body) was added. A third group of mice received the mixture of curcumin and olive oil without fluoridated water, and a fourth group of mice served as controls.

Prior to conducting this study, the researchers involved had spent nearly a decade studying the various ways in which fluoride causes neurodegenerative damages and other harmful changes in the brains of mammals. In doing so, they found that fluoride causes a significant increase in the oxidation of the brain's fatty tissues and cells (a process known as *lipid peroxidation,* or LPO), and also increases the growth and spread of neurodegenerative cells in the brain's hippocampus region and cerebral cortex. One of the markers for, or indicators of, lipid peroxidation is called malondialdehyde, or MDA. MDA naturally occurs as a result of lipid peroxidation and acts as both a carcinogen and a mutagen.

In the mice group that consumed fluoridated water alone, levels of MDA were significantly elevated, as was overall lipid peroxidation. As the researchers noted, a single daily dose of fluoride via the water resulted in "highly significant increases in the LPO as well as neurodegenerative changes in neuron cell bodies of selected hippocampal regions" in the brains of the mice. By contrast, in the mice group that consumed both fluoridated water and the curcumin/olive oil mixture it was found that "supplementation with curcumin significantly reduce the toxic effect of F[luoride] to near normal levels by augmenting the antioxidant defense through [curcumin's] scavenging property." As a result, the researchers concluded that curcumin offers important therapeutic benefits in protecting against brain cell damage and degeneration that fluoride is known to cause.

To further protect against exposure to fluoride in water, many people choose to use water filters, yet most of them do not filter out fluoride. Therefore, if you choose to use a water filter, research product brands beforehand and consider contacting the manufacturer if you have any questions. Also be aware that fluoridated water can be absorbed by your body when you shower or bathe, so you might consider installing an overall home water filtration system if you can afford it, such as a reverse osmosis filtration system. Such systems typically remove between 90 to 95 percent of fluoride in municipal tap water.

You can also consider buying and using a water distiller. The distillation process effectively removes fluoride and a host of other contaminants from water that are harmful to your health. In addition, avoid fluoridated toothpastes and dental products, as well as all processed food and commercial teas and other beverages.

CONCLUSION

You now have a much greater understanding of the factors that can affect the health of your brain, and you also are aware of how and why both turmeric and curcumin can play vital roles in helping to keep your brain, and therefore you, healthy throughout your life. I encourage you to work with your physician to address and minimize the impact of the risk factors you learned about in this chapter, and to start using turmeric to spice up your meals.

For added benefit, you can also consider taking a daily curcumin supplement. You will find guidelines on how to do so and what to look for when choosing such supplements in Chapter 10. In the next chapter, you will discover the promise that both turmeric and curcumin have for preventing and helping to treat another most serious and greatly feared disease—cancer.

4

A Novel Cancer Fighter

"You have cancer."

For most people, those are perhaps the most frightening words in the English language. That's because they view a diagnosis of cancer as being akin to being handed a death sentence. Although advances continue be made in the "war on cancer," such a view is not unfounded. Overall, the medical establishment's record of success when it comes to treating most forms of cancer still remains abysmal. This is especially true in cases where cancer has metastasized, meaning after it has spread from its original tumor site to other organs and tissues. Therefore, doing all that you can to prevent cancer is vitally important. In this chapter, you will learn how turmeric's active ingredient, curcumin, can help you do so.

FAST FACTS ABOUT CANCER

Cancer is a disease in which certain cells in the body stop functioning and maturing properly. As the normal cycle of cell creation and death is interrupted, these newly mutated cancer cells begin multiplying uncontrollably, no longer operating as an integrated and harmonious part of the body. They also develop their own network of blood vessels to siphon nourishment away from the body's blood supply. This process, if unchecked, will eventually lead to the formation of a cancerous tumor. As the abnormal cells often migrate into and circulate within the bloodstream, the cancer can also spread to other parts of the body. This process, known as *metastasis,* can cause the formation of more tumors and further sap the body's energy supply, weakening and eventually poisoning the patient with toxic byproducts.

Every cell in the human body has the ability to turn cancerous, and many do so on a daily basis. Normally, the immune system is able to protect the body by destroying these cells or reprogramming them back to normal functioning. If the body's defense systems have been damaged, however, this process cannot happen, allowing the cancer to establish itself.

There is no single cause of cancer. Instead, many interdependent factors contribute to its development, which is one of the reasons why cancer is so difficult to successfully treat. Each type of cancer can be caused by a variety of factors, ranging from air pollution and tobacco smoke, to environmental radiation and industrial chemicals such as asbestos, benzene, and vinyl chloride, to naturally occurring substances such as aflatoxins (toxins produced by fungus commonly found in peanuts, corn, milk, and other foods), as well as the body's own production of free radicals.

Though the causes of cancer are still being debated, science is much closer today to understanding the fundamental factors involved in the process. For some time, it has been clear that tumors arise as a result of a series of changes or rearrangements of information coded in the DNA within single cells. The factors that initiate cancer are known as *triggers* or *carcinogens*. Carcinogens interact directly with cellular DNA to disrupt its normal functioning, thereby triggering the cell damage that leads to cells becoming cancerous.

The incidence of cancer has increased from the beginning of the twentieth century, when it struck three percent of the population, to the present day, when 50 percent of men and over 40 percent of women are expected to develop it. Cancer is the second leading cause of death in the United States, behind only heart disease, and has actually overtaken heart disease as the top cause of death for all people below the age of eighty-five.

According to the Centers for Disease Control and Prevention (CDC), over 600,000 Americans die from cancer each year. And data collected by the National Cancer Institute (NCI) reveals that nearly 1.7 million other Americans are diagnosed with cancer every year.

The NCI lists the most common types of cancer in the United States as:

- bladder cancer
- breast cancer
- colon and rectum cancer
- endometrial cancer
- kidney and renal pelvis cancer
- leukemia
- lung and bronchus cancer
- melanoma of the skin
- non-Hodgkin's lymphoma
- pancreatic cancer
- prostate cancer
- thyroid cancer

According to the American Cancer Society, the incidence of rare types of cancer is on the rise, with approximately 13 percent of all cancers diagnosed in American adults ages twenty or older now being rare types of cancers.

Many new discoveries and treatment options have emerged since the "war on cancer" was officially declared by President Nixon in 1971, at which time only one out of every ten Americans developed cancer. Yet overall survival rates, with the exception of a few select types of cancer, are not much better today than they were then.

Because cancer remains so difficult to treat, prevention and regular screening tests to detect it early are the two most important steps you can take to protect yourself. Early detection of cancer can dramatically improve treatment outcomes. Preventive measures involve eating a healthy diet of organic foods with an emphasis on fiber-rich foods and an abundant intake of fresh fruits and vegetables each day. Minimizing your exposure to environmental toxins, avoiding exposure to secondhand smoke, managing stress, getting adequate sleep, and supplementing your diet with nutritional supplements, herbs, and spices have all been shown to act as natural cancer-fighters.

Topping the list of such spices is turmeric, while curcumin in supplement form has also been shown by research to provide multiple potent anti-cancer benefits.

KNOW THE SIGNS AND SYMPTOMS OF CANCER

Recognizing the early warning signs and symptoms of cancer can help ensure an early diagnosis. This makes it potentially easier to treat cancer before it has *metastasized* (spread to other areas of the body). Cancer that is detected early typically has not yet had the opportunity to deplete the body of its disease-fighting resources, and is therefore far more likely to respond to treatment and result in remission, regardless of which category it belongs to.

Early Warning Signs

What follows are the most common early warning signs, or initial symptoms, of cancer. If you experience any one of the following symptoms, seek immediate medical attention so that you can be properly screened for cancer.

Lumps of Thickening in Breast or Testicle Tissues

Since breast and testicular cancer have increasingly shown signs of developing earlier, all men and women above the age of twenty-five should regularly (at least once a month) examine themselves for telltale signs of cancer of the breasts and testicles. By gently yet firmly pressing into the breasts, women are often able to detect lumps or thickening breast tissue that can be a sign of breast cancer. In a similar fashion, men can massage their testicles, being on the lookout for any noticeable changes in the way they feel.

Changes in Warts or Moles

Warts or moles that begin to change appearance can be a sign of various types of skin cancer, such as melanoma or squamous carcinoma. One indication that skin cancer might be developing is bleeding that occurs in warts and moles. Change in wart or mole size is another common indicator. In addition, the appearance of chronic pimples or patches of dry, scaly skin are other warning signs, as is skin that becomes inflamed or ulcerated. Sores that are slow to heal are another indicator, as are chronic sores in the mouth.

Persistent Sore Throat

A chronic sore throat can be a potential indicator that cancer is developing in the esophagus, larynx, or pharynx. Other early warning signs of throat cancer include persistent hoarseness, lumps in the throat, and difficulty swallowing.

Changes in Bowel and Bladder Habits

Any noticeable and persistent change in your bowel movements or in the way you urinate can be an indication of cancer in the genitourinary tract (bladder, prostate, and testicular cancer), or in the gastrointestinal tract (colon or stomach cancer). Such changes include unexplained constipation or diarrhea, blood in the urine or stool, pain during urination and elimination, difficulty urinating or passing stool, abdominal pain, and stools that are dark and resemble tar.

Coughing Blood/Persistent Coughing

Persistent coughing and coughing up of blood can be signs of lung cancer, as well as other types of cancer, especially in people who smoke.

Chronic Digestion Problems

The following digestive symptoms can all be indications of cancer: abdominal pain, bloating of the stomach or abdomen, chronic heartburn or indigestion, nausea, and loss of appetite. Chronic flatulence is another potential early warning sign, as is a persistent "growling" stomach.

Unexplained Weight Loss

Any sudden and unexplained loss of weight should immediately be brought to the attention of your doctor.

Persistent Fatigue and Feelings of Exhaustion

Ongoing loss of energy or chronic fatigue can be signs that cancer is present and beginning to spread.

Abnormal Vaginal Discharges or Bleeding

These signs can be indications of cervical, ovarian, or vaginal cancer.

Cancer Symptoms by Type

Cancer can manifest itself in many different ways throughout your body. There are many symptoms associated with cancer, and they can vary considerably depending on the kind of cancer (or cancers) in question. Below are some of the indicators and symptoms you or a loved one may experience if afflicted.

Relying on self-care screening methods alone is usually not enough to detect cancer, however. People forty years or older, as well as anyone with a family history of cancer, should consider receiving professional screening tests on an annual basis.

Bladder Cancer Symptoms

Early indicators of bladder cancer include blood in the urine, rust-colored urine, pain or burning sensations during urination, frequent need to urinate, difficulty urinating, and pus-filled urine.

Bone Cancer (Sarcoma) Symptoms

Symptoms of bone cancer, or sarcoma, consist of unexplained weakness in areas of the musculoskeletal system, unexplained pains in and around areas of the bones, and increased susceptibility to fractures.

Breast Cancer Symptoms

Lumps in the breast or thickening breast tissue, nipple discharge, retraction of the nipple, dimpling of breast tissue, reddened breast skin tissue, swollen breasts, sensation of heat in the breasts, and swelling in the lymph nodes beneath the armpits are all signs of breast cancer.

Colon or Rectal Cancer Symptoms

Early warning signs of cancer in the colon or rectum include blood in the stools, bleeding from the rectum, dark and tarry stools, abdominal pains and cramping, unexplained constipation or diarrhea, alternating constipation and diarrhea, unexplained weight loss, loss of appetite, unexplained fatigue, and poor skin pallor.

Kidney Cancer Symptoms

Kidney cancer may be present if you experience symptoms such as blood in the urine, dull aches or pains in the lower back or on the sides of the abdomen, lumps or swelling in the kidney area of the abdomen or lower back, unexplained elevations in blood pressure levels, or unexplained abnormalities in red blood cell count.

Leukemia Symptoms

Signs and symptoms associated with leukemia are unexplained weakness or fatigue, pale skin, unexplained fever, flu-like symptoms, prolonged bleeding, unexplained bruising, enlarged lymph nodes, swollen spleen or liver, frequent infections, unexplained bone or joint pain, unexplained weight loss, and night sweats.

Lung Cancer Symptoms

Lung cancer typically presents itself as symptoms including persistent coughing or wheezing, constant chest pain, continual lung congestion, swollen lymph nodes in the neck, and blood produced upon coughing.

Melanoma (Skin Cancer) Symptoms

Changes in skin tone and texture, changes in the size, shape, or color of moles, and unexplained bleeding from the skin are all indicators of skin cancer, or melanoma of the skin.

Non-Hodgkin's Lymphoma Symptoms

Non-Hodgkin's lymphoma manifests itself as swelling (without pain) of the lymph nodes in the neck, armpits, or groin; persistent fever; persistent fatigue; unexplained weight loss; unexplained skin rashes or itching; small lumps in the skin; bone pain; and swelling in the liver, spleen, or areas of the abdomen.

Oral (Lip, Mouth, or Throat) Cancer Symptoms

Oral cancer may present itself as lumps or sore spots in the mouth, pain while eating or drinking, persistent ulcers on the lip, tongue or inside the mouth, difficulty swallowing, oral pain, loosening teeth, bleeding in the mouth, blood produced by coughing, or persistent bad breath.

Ovarian Cancer Symptoms

Symptoms of ovarian cancer include abdominal swelling, unexplained vaginal bleeding or discharge, and persistent and unexplained digestive problems.

Pancreatic Cancer Symptoms

Persistent pain in the upper abdomen, unexplained weight loss, persistent pain in the mid-back and center of the back, loss of appetite, sudden inability to properly digest/tolerate fatty foods, yellow skin tone (jaundice), abdominal swelling, and swelling of the liver and spleen are all indicators of cancer of the pancreas.

Prostate Cancer Symptoms

Indicators of prostate cancer include difficulty urinating, pain or burning sensations upon urination, frequent need to urinate, incomplete urination, blood in the urine, pain in the area of the bladder, and dull, persistent aching in the area of the pelvis and lower back.

Uterine Cancer (Cancer of the Uterus) Symptoms

Approximately 70 to 75 percent of all cases of uterine cancer occur after menopause. Symptoms include vaginal bleeding or discharge after menopause, painful urination, collection of fluids in the uterus, pain during intercourse, and persistent pains in the area of the pelvis.

HOW CURCUMIN PROTECTS AGAINST CANCER

A growing body of studies, which first began more than fifty years ago, continues to find that curcumin holds potent anticancer benefits. In fact, curcumin's promise as an anticancer agent is so powerful that in 2003, scientists from the famed M.D. Anderson Cancer Center in Texas wrote, "Extensive research over the last fifty years has indicated this polyphenol [curcumin] can both prevent and treat cancer . . . [and] can suppress tumor initiation, promotion, and metastasis."

The anti-cancer benefits of curcumin are primarily due to its ability to protect against free radical damage and inflammation, increase cellular glutathione levels, induce normal cell death (apoptosis), inhibit tumor growth, inhibit cancer cells from developing their own network of blood vessels that supply nutrient fuel for cancer cells and tumors (angiogenesis), increase the activity of biotransformation enzymes that help eliminate biologically active carcinogens, and block estrogen-mimicking chemicals.

Protection Against Free Radical Damage

Free radical damage is caused by excessive oxidation of cells and tissues. The oxidizing effects of free radicals harm cellular DNA and have been shown to contribute to numerous diseases, including cancer. As we have already discussed, curcumin acts as a potent antioxidant that can protect against free radicals. This has been demonstrated in a number of cancer studies, including studies that have shown that curcumin inhibits the generation of tumor-causing effects of reactive oxygen species (ROS), including in white blood cells (leukocytes) which are part of the body's immune system. Healthy immune function is essential for protecting against cancer.

Defense Against ROS and Oxidative Damage

Additional research has shown that curcumin is an effective scavenger of reactive nitrogen species, which can also cause cancer. Other studies have demonstrated curcumin's protective effects against oxidative damage to the skin. Still other studies have demonstrated curcumin's ability to protect against both cellular DNA damage caused by oxidation, and the oxidation of healthy fats (*lipid peroxidation*), both of which can result in the formation of cancer cells.

Prevention of Chronic Inflammation

As you now know, curcumin also has potent anti-inflammatory properties. Chronic inflammation is a primary contributing cause of cancer. Curcumin protects against inflammation, and therefore cancer, in a number of ways. First, curcumin inhibits the activation of *nuclear factor-kappaB* (NF-κB), which can trigger the expression of pro-inflammatory genes. Second, curcumin inhibits the expression of *cyclooxygenase-2* (COX-2) and *5-lypoxygenase* (5-LOX), two enzymes involved in inflammation. Additionally, curcumin binds to 5-LOX to directly inhibit its activity. These genes and enzymes, when unchecked, can play a role in the development and spread of cancer. Research also shows that curcumin inhibits the expression of various cell surface adhesion molecules, cytokines, and chemokines, all of which are directly related to inflammation and can ultimately lead to healthy, normal cells in the body becoming cancerous.

Production of Glutathione

Curcumin's ability to increase cellular glutathione levels is another significant health benefit. Glutathione is an important antioxidant that plays a critical role in supporting cellular adaptation to stress. The better cells are able to resist such stress, the more resistant they are to cancer. Research has shown that curcumin elevates cellular glutathione levels through its ability to enhance the gene expression of *glutamate cysteine ligase* (GCL), an enzyme involved in glutathione synthesis.

Induction of Apoptosis

Curcumin's potential for inducing *apoptosis* (normal cell death) is also important. Healthy cells pass through a sequence of stages each time that they divide. These stages are known as a cell cycle, and each stage must be passed through before a healthy cell can divide again. Under normal circumstances, when DNA damage occurs, the cell cycle is arrested so that DNA can be repaired. If repair is not possible, then mechanisms are activated within the cell that cause its death.

If this process becomes defective, however, cells do not die. Instead, they may mutate, eventually to the point where they turn cancerous. Inducing apoptosis is an important goal in the treatment of cancer, and studies of various cancer cell lines grown in culture have demonstrated that curcumin has the potential to achieve this. It does this in a variety of ways, including inhibiting cell-signaling pathways that, if not suppressed, can lead to unnatural cell division.

Interruption of Angiogenesis

In addition to inducing apoptosis, cancer specialists also seek to interrupt the process known as *angiogenesis*. Angiogenesis is a process that results in cancer cells and tumors developing their own network of blood vessels, through which they feed and grow. Once this angiogenic network develops, cancer cells and tumors can divert vital nutrients from the rest of the body to weaken it and further compromise immune function. In addition, as angiogenesis progresses and cancer cells spread, they invade normal tissues via enzymes called *matrix metalloproteinases* (MMP). Cell culture studies have shown that curcumin inhibits the activity of MMP. Cell culture and animal studies have also shown that curcumin also inhibits angiogenesis directly.

Increased Activity of Biotransformation Enzymes

Curcumin has beneficial effects on biotransformation enzymes. This class of enzymes plays an important role in helping the body process all of the various chemical compounds that we are exposed to daily, including the chemicals in nutritional supplements, pharmaceutical drugs, and environmental toxins. Biotransformation enzymes are critical for the elimination of various carcinogens from the body. Cell culture and animal studies have demonstrated that curcumin can increase the activity of these cancer-fighting enzymes, thereby enhancing their ability to eliminate carcinogens.

Blockage of Estrogen-Mimicking Chemicals

Curcumin blocks health-damaging chemicals from entering cells, something that sets it apart from most other natural anticancer compounds. Curcumin is especially effective in preventing estrogen-mimicking chemicals, such as DDT, dioxin, chlordane, and endosulfane, from penetrating cells. It does this by its ability to pass through a cell receptor called *aryl hydrocarbon*, which acts as a cellular doorway. Both estrogen and the chemicals that mimic it also enter cells through aryl hydrocarbon receptors. Because curcumin can compete with them for the receptor, it has the ability to block their access into cells, thus preventing them from becoming damaged and turning cancerous.

Like estrogen itself, estrogen-mimicking chemicals promote the growth and spread of breast cancer. One study of human breast cancer cells showed that curcumin reversed the growth of breast cancer cells caused by 17b-estradiol by 98 percent. The same study also found that curcumin reversed breast cancer cell growth caused by DDT by 75 percent.

Additional research showed that curcumin reversed the growth of breast cancer cell growth caused by chlordane and endosulfane, both of which also mimic estrogen, by 90 percent. When combined with the soy-derived compound genistein, curcumin resulted in a 100 percent halt to cancer cell growth. Curcumin also has the ability to block other carcinogenic chemicals from entering inside cells, thereby reducing the incidence of cancer. For example, in a study with mice treated with the toxin diethylnitrosamine, curcumin reduced the percentage of mice that developed cancer from 100 percent to 38 percent, and reduced the formation of tumors by 81 percent.

Stopping Infections

Research has also found that curcumin also helps prevent and stop the spread of bacterial, fungal, and viral infections that can also trigger cancer and make it worse because of how these infectious agents weaken the body's immune system.

Multi-Targeted Therapies

Even more exciting, studies have also found that curcumin's mechanisms of actions in the body are in many ways similar to various classes of anticancer drugs, including recently discovered tumor necrosis factor blocking drugs such as Humira, Remicade, and Enbrel; vascular endothelial cell growth factor blocking drugs such as Avastin; human epidermal growth factor receptor blocking drugs such as Erbitux, Erlotinib, and Geftinib; and HER2 blocking drugs such as Herceptin. Cancer researchers and physicians today increasingly employ multi-targeted therapies that combine these different classes of drugs to improve cancer outcomes. Curcumin, studies demonstrate, offers many of these same multi-targeted benefits.

Given all of the above mechanisms of actions it possesses, you can understand why researchers are so excited about curcumin's use as a natural anticancer agent. Now let's look at curcumin's benefits for protecting against specific types of cancer.

CURCUMIN'S WIDE SCOPE OF DEFENSE

Curcumin has proven itself to be a strong defense against many different types of cancers, including brain cancer, breast cancer, prostate cancer, and more. Research shows that curcumin not only protects against the development of cancer, but also works to help reverse it.

Brain Cancer

A number of studies highlight curcumin's promise for preventing and helping to treat brain cancer, which is one of the most challenging types of cancer. Research with mice has shown, for example, that because curcumin is capable of crossing the blood-brain barrier without causing harm to healthy brain cells, it has the ability to block the formation of brain neuroblastoma tumors while also eliminating neuroblastoma cells by inducing apoptosis. This study builds on previous research of human neuroblastoma cell lines, which showed that curcumin, in combination with resveratrol, a compound derived from wine and grapes, also induces apoptosis in neuroblastoma cells. *Neuroblastoma* is a particularly aggressive form of brain cancer that affects the peripheral nervous system and primarily strikes in childhood.

Studies have demonstrated that curcumin can also provide preventive and therapeutic benefit for *glioblastoma,* another type of brain cancer that affects the glial cells of the brain and spinal cord, forming tumors known as *gliomas.* The most common form of gliomas are astrocystomas, which develop from star-shaped cells known as *astrocytes.* The spread of these types of tumors is promoted by the NF-kappaB protein. In a study of human astrocytoma cell lines, curcumin was shown to inhibit NF-kappaB in five different types of astrocytoma cell lines. It also promoted apoptosis in these cultured cells. Another study showed that curcumin inhibited the growth and induced the death of human brain glioblastoma multiforme 8401 (GBM 8401) cells.

Breast Cancer

In addition to its proven ability to prevent estrogen-mimicking carcinogens from passing inside cells, curcumin can protect against breast cancer in other ways, including enhancing the immune system's ability to detect and attack breast cancer cells.

One challenging characteristic of cancer tumors is that they can "hide" from the immune system, thereby eluding natural killer (NK) cells that play a primary role in destroying them. Tumors do this by secreting substances known as *exosomes*. Exosomes contain proteins that can fuse with immune cells and inhibit NK cell activity. Research with mouse breast tumor cells shows that curcumin can reverse the ability of exosomes to suppress NK cells' immune benefits. Another study involving rats showed that curcumin can prevent breast tissues from becoming cancerous due to radiation exposure. Given the radiation that women are exposed to each time they receive a mammogram, this finding suggests that curcumin could be beneficial before, during, and after mammography exams.

Curcumin also helps to control the growth of human breast cancer cells even when they are drug-resistant. Breast cancer cells grow and spread in part because of the release of a substance called *arachidonate acid* (AA) by the enzyme *phospholipase A2*. As AA is released, it causes breast cancer cells to grow and spread. In a study of cultured human breast cancer cells, curcumin blocked the spread of the cancerous cells by altering AA metabolism. This was true even in breast cancer cells that had proven to be resistant to cancer drugs. Curcumin used in combination with *xanthorrhizol*, another compound found in turmeric, induces apoptosis of human breast cancer cells, as well.

One of the most significant studies of curcumin's breast cancer benefits was published in 2009. In that study, the researchers examined the effects of curcumin in a specific type of breast cancer known as triple negative breast cancer. This type of breast cancer is very difficult to treat, and when it recurs, conventional medicine has a poor record of successfully treating it. The study showed that curcumin caused the death of triple negative cancer cells by damaging their DNA, and preventing them from spreading.

Curcumin achieved these effects through its ability to modulate the gene known as breast cancer 1, early onset (BRCA1). BRCA1 belongs to a class of genes known as *tumor suppressor genes*. The protein produced from the BRCA1 gene helps prevent cells from growing and dividing too rapidly, or in an uncontrolled way. Researchers have identified more than 1,000 mutations in the BRCA1 gene, many of which are associated with an increased risk of cancer, especially breast cancer. This study indicated that curcumin helps BRCA1 maintain its integrity.

Colon Cancer

Curcumin has particular promise in preventing and treating colon cancer, in part due to how well curcumin is absorbed by both healthy and malignant cells and tissues of the colon and overall gastrointestinal tract. This was demonstrated in a study of patients with advanced colorectal cancer who took 3.6 grams of curcumin orally for seven days. At the end of that period, measurable amounts of curcumin were found in both healthy and cancerous tissues.

Both in vitro (laboratory) studies and phase I human clinical trials have demonstrated curcumin's ability to prevent colon cancer, and the phase I studies also found that curcumin is both safe and well tolerated by cancer patients, even at doses as high as eight grams per day. Curcumin helps to prevent and treat colon cancer in various ways. Its preventative properties are primarily due to its antioxidant and anti-inflammatory properties, while therapeutically it checks the spread of colon cancer cells, inducing their death and altering the expression of various genes involved in their development. In addition, curcumin inhibits *neurotenion,* a gastrointestinal hormone that acts as a potent trigger in inducing tumor cell expression in both colon and pancreatic cancer, and in triggering the spread of human colon cancer cells. Both animal and human cell line studies have shown that curcumin also targets and inhibits the activity of the cancer trigger protein complex *proteasome,* leading to increased colon cancer cell death and decreased tumor growth. Other research has shown that curcumin inhibits cell-signaling that can otherwise trigger the spread of colon cancer cells.

One of the most exciting studies about curcumin as a treatment for colon cancer revealed that it is effective at preventing the emergence of cancer stem cells (CSCs), both alone and when used in conjunction with chemotherapy drugs. The success of such drugs when used alone can be limited in part due to CSCs, which are highly resistant to chemotherapy. In this study, colon cancer CSCs that had proven to be resistant to the colon cancer drug FOLFOX were treated with curcumin alone, and with a combination of curcumin and FOLFOX. In both cases, the researchers observed a significant reduction in colon CSCs, leading to the disintegration of colon cancer cell colonies. This result has not been achieved against colon CSCs using FOLFOX alone and represents a promising new development in the effective treatment for recurring colon cancer.

Prostate Cancer

Prostate cancer is another area for which curcumin offers help. Prostate cancer is the number one type of cancer to strike men in the Western world. In contrast, in Asian countries in which curcumin-rich turmeric is commonly used as a spice, the incidence of prostate cancer is relatively low. Researchers have found that curcumin and turmeric in the diet suppresses prostate tumor development because of their antioxidant properties, and their ability to inhibit arachidonic acid metabolism, modulate cell signaling pathways, and inhibit hormone and growth factor activity and oncogene expression. (Oncogenes cause normal cells in the body to transfrom in cancer cells.) Curcumin's ability in these areas is on par with genestein, a soybean-derived product that is commonly used by many physicians to help prevent and treat prostate cancer.

Curcumin also slows the rate at which hormone-responsive prostate cancer cells become resistant to hormonal therapy, and increases the sensitivity of these cells to chemotherapy. In addition, curcumin enhances the ability of a protein known as *TNF-related apoptosis inducing ligand* (TRAIL) to induce apoptosis in prostate cancer cells. The TRAIL protein is one of the compounds the body uses to target and kill prostate cancer cells. It is significantly altered when prostate cancer develops, and as a result, its ability to induce apoptosis on its own is severely reduced.

Curcumin can also inhibit the growth and spread of prostate cancer cells by down-regulating the androgen and epidermal growth factor receptors associated with them. Curcumin's various anticancer mechanisms of action also enhance the effects of radiation therapy for prostate cancer. Other research has demonstrated that curcumin's protective antioxidant effects against prostate cancer are more potent than garlic, devil's claw, and fish oil, making it an excellent dietary source of protection.

Other Types of Cancer

Numerous studies indicate that curcumin offers benefits for other types of cancer, as well. As researchers continue to investigate curcumin's anticancer properties, it is likely that the range of cancers for which it may be helpful will grow.

Bladder Cancer

Curcumin has been shown to decrease the expression of *specificity protein transcription factors* (Sp proteins) that play a role in the development and spread of bladder cancer. Specifically, curcumin has been shown to increase apoptosis of bladder cancer cells and decrease their ability to achieve angiogenesis. Research has also shown that curcumin administered directly into the bladder region following surgery for bladder cancer can help prevent its recurrence.

Leukemia

Curcumin also induces apoptosis in, and inhibits the spread of, human leukemia cells. Curcumin combined with green tea also has value for treating B-chronic lymphocytic leukemia due to their shared ability to induce apoptosis. Similar research shows that curcumin inhibits the spread of human B-cell non-Hodgkin's lymphoma cells without harming normal blood cells.

Liver Cancer

A number of animal studies show that curcumin also protects against liver cancer due to its ability to inhibit the actions of carcinogens known to trigger the development of liver cancer cells. Curcumin may also have benefit as a treatment for pituitary cancer. A study of rats demonstrated that curcumin inhibits the growth of pituitary cancer cells, kills them, and decreases the production and release of prolactin and growth hormone 3 (GH3), two hormones that are associated with pituitary cancer.

Pancreatic Cancer

Curcumin also offers promise for pancreatic cancer. Researchers investigating curcumin's effects on human pancreatic cancer cell lines found that it can arrest their cell cycle and induce them to die. Additionally, curcumin combined with isoflavone, another natural compound derived from soy, works synergistically to improve the ability of both compounds to inhibit the growth of pancreatic cancer cells and induce apoptosis. Additional research has shown that drug analogs of curcumin, known as FLLL11 and FLLL12, are also effective in suppressing the growth activity of human pancreatic cells.

Skin Cancer

Skin cancer is another area for which curcumin can be beneficial. It inhibits squamous cell cancer growth in the head and neck, and the growth and spread of tumors when applied topically to squamous cell cancer grafts. Curcumin has also been shown to have benefit for melanoma. Research with mice found that curcumin triggers a process known as *endoplasmic reticulum* (ER) stress. When prolonged, ER stress can lead to programmed cell death of melanoma cells. A study of human melanoma cell lines has also shown that curcumin can induce the death of melanoma cells. Another mouse study demonstrated that curcumin also enhances the effects of the chemotherapy drugs Thalomid (*thalidomide*) and Velcade (*bortezombib*), both of which are used as treatments for multiple myeloma, by inhibiting the ability of myeloma cells to develop resistance to these drugs.

How Curcumin Helped
a Dying Woman Beat Myeloma

As I was gathering research in preparation to writing this book, I came across a news article about how curcumin was responsible for a woman's remarkable recovery from myeloma. Myeloma is a type of blood cancer that is caused when white blood cells that are produced in the body's bone marrow begin to multiply uncontrollably, while at the same time stop producing antibodies the body requires to fight infections. Symptoms of myeloma include bone and nerve damage, excruciating pain, and intense fatigue. Although its progression can be slowed by various cancer drugs, overall myeloma is considered incurable, and the majority of people who are afflicted by it typically die within five years or less of their diagnoses. Were it not for curcumin, the woman profiled in the article would likely have been one of them.

The woman's name is Dieneke Ferguson. She lives in London, England and was sixty-seven at the time the article was written. She was first diagnosed with myeloma in 2007. In order to treat it, she underwent three rounds of chemotherapy, as well as four stem cell transplants. "I have been on all sorts of toxic drugs and the side-effects were terrifying," Ferguson said in the article. "At one point I lost my memory for three days, and in 2008, two of the vertebrae in my spine collapsed so I couldn't walk. They injected some kind of concrete into my spine to keep it stable."

All of Ferguson's treatments proved unsuccessful. After experiencing a temporary stabilization of her condition, she suffered a relapse, and by 2012 both she and her doctors felt there was little hope that her life could be saved. That was when Ferguson came across mention of curcumin as a possible aid for cancer patients in an Internet support group. She decided to try it because, she says, "I had nothing to lose. All my options were exhausted, and there was nothing else I could do. There was just too much cancer."

To her doctors' surprise, it worked. Five years after she first began taking a curcumin supplement on a daily basis, during which time she received no further conventional medical treatments, her cancer cell count at the time the article appeared was negligible. "When you review her chart, there's no alternative explanation [for her recovery] other than we're seeing a response to curcumin," states Jamie Cavanagh, MD, a professor of blood diseases and one of Ferguson's oncologists at St. Bartholomew's Hospital in London. Cavanagh co-authored a paper about Ferguson's recovery in the *British Medical Journal* (BMJ) because of how extraordinary he considers it to be.

"Curcumin is a strong anti-inflammatory agent and chronic inflammation is the precursor of 99 percent of all cancers," Angus Dalgleish, a professor of cancer at St. George's Hospital in South London, was quoted as saying in the article. "Taking regular anti-inflammatory agents such as aspirin is known to reduce the risk of colon cancer by around 30 percent and have an impact on the incidence of others too, but lack of funding for research has prevented most [people] from benefiting from curcumin."

The article reported that Ferguson continues to take a curcumin supplement every day at a daily dose of eight grams in tablet form, which is the equivalent of two teaspoons of pure, powdered curcumin, an amount that is not possible to obtain from turmeric spice alone.

In summarizing her case history, Dr. Cavanagh and his co-authors of the BMJ report wrote, "The fact that our patient, who had advanced stage disease and was effectively salvaged while exclusively on curcumin, suggests a potential antimyeloma effect of curcumin. She continues to take daily curcumin and remains in a very satisfactory condition with good quality of life. This case provides further evidence of the potential benefit for curcumin in myeloma. We would recommend further evaluation of curcumin in myeloma patients in the context of a clinical trial."

STEPS YOU CAN TAKE
TO LOWER YOUR RISK FOR CANCER

It's wisely been said that the best way to treat cancer is to prevent it from developing in the first place. Although cancer is often considered to be a genetic disease, meaning that it occurs if a person is born with various oncogenes, the truth is that the presence of oncogenes in the body, of themselves, matter far less than whether or not they are "turned on" or activated. Scientists now know that the primary way in which this activation occurs is through our dietary and lifestyle choices, our exposure to environmental toxins, and the degree to which we experience chronic stress and debilitating emotions. And research confirms that nearly 40 percent of all cases of cancer are caused by poor lifestyle choices. This means that correcting these choices has the potential to reduce cancer rates by nearly 40 percent as well.

For all of its potent anticancer properties, curcumin is hardly a "magic bullet" for protecting against cancer. No such magic bullet exists. However, there is much that you can do on your own to significantly reduce your risk of ever developing cancer. Some of the most vital steps you can take are as follows:

Diet

Poor diet is a significant risk factor for cancer because of nutritional deficiencies and lack of cancer-protecting fiber it results in. The likelihood of developing colon or rectal cancer, lung cancer, or throat cancers of the oral cavity, larynx, or pharynx is especially increased by poor diet.

To improve your diet, try to consume at least seven to nine servings of fresh, fiber-rich, non-starchy vegetables each day, along with three to five servings of fresh fruit. Dark, leafy green vegetables, as well as cruciferous vegetables such as broccoli, cauliflower, or Brussels sprouts are particularly good choices, along with garlic and onions, as are berries, oranges, and other citrus fruits. Ideally, try to purchase only organic fruits and vegetables. Fruits should be eaten uncooked, while non-starchy vegetables are best consumed raw or lightly steamed so as to prevent the wide array of nutrients and enzymes they contain from being destroyed by heat. Seeds, nuts, and wild-caught fish such as sardines and salmon are also good food choices.

Limit your overall consumption of carbohydrate foods, especially breads, pasta, and other wheat products, since a low-carb diet in conjunction with a moderate to high supply of healthy fats has been shown to have the potential to lower cancer risk. Also avoid using unsaturated and polyunsaturated oils, all of which can cause chronic inflammation. Extra virgin olive oil is permissible, but for cooking purposes consider unrefined, cold-pressed coconut oil instead.

Avoid sugar and simple carbohydrates as much as possible, since they both breakdown into glucose, which is cancer's primary fuel. Also avoid all processed meats and limit your weekly red meat intake. Focus instead on lean, free-range poultry or lamb. Also be sure to consume adequate amounts of pure, filtered water each day, and avoid sodas and commercial fruit juices and nonherbal teas. Herbal teas, on the other hand, are advised, as is certified organic green tea, which is known to provide important anticancer benefits.

Alcohol

Aside from no more than one or two glasses of red wine or beer each day, alcoholic beverages should be avoided altogether, as regular alcohol consumption can increase the risk for cancer, especially breast, colon, liver, stomach, and throat cancers. But even moderate intake of beer or wine cannot be guaranteed to be completely safe, so you may want to avoid even those beverages altogether.

Smoking

Cigarette smoking remains one of the greatest risk factors for cancer, especially, but not limited to, lung cancer. Although the incidence of lung cancer among nonsmokers continues to rise, smoking increases that risk by as much as 500 percent. If you smoke, get help so that you can quit. Chronic exposure to secondhand smoke can also increase your cancer risk, and should also be avoided.

Exercise

Physical inactivity also increases the risk for cancer, especially, breast, colon, and endometrial cancer. Intense regular exercise is not necessary to reduce this risk, however. Research shows that as little as three to five hours per week of moderate exercise, such as walking or bicycling, is all that is necessary to lower your cancer risk.

Maintaining a Healthy Weight

Sadly, in the past few decades the United States has become an obese nation. With certain exceptions, being unhealthily overweight or obese is primarily the result of self-inflicted lifestyle choices. Being overweight increases the risk of many types of cancer, as well as many other serious degenerative diseases, including heart disease, stroke, diabetes, and Alzheimer's disease and dementia. If you are overweight and want to reduce your risk of cancer, you must work with your doctor to do all you can to reduce your weight safely and permanently.

Sleep

Nightly healthy, deep, adequate sleep is also essential for helping to maintain your overall health, and thus reducing your risk for cancer. If you suffer from poor sleep, speak with your doctor to improve your sleep without resorting to sleeping pills. Also do your best to obtain at least seven to eight hours of sleep each night. Doing so will help your body to more effectively repair and restore itself, as well as reducing stress and improving your mood. It will also provide you with more energy throughout the day.

Stress Management

Chronic stress, as well as unresolved mental and emotional issues, all weaken the body's immune system and thus can greatly increase the risk for cancer, as well as many other diseases. If you suffer from chronic stress or lingering mental or emotional issues, consider working with a holistically-oriented physician or counselor (someone whose first instinct is not to prescribe dangerous antidepressants or other drugs) to address these problems. There is also much that you can do on your own to reduce stress, such as socializing with friends and family members whose company you enjoy, sharing your concerns with someone you trust, spending time in nature, meditating, making time on a regular basis to engage in hobbies or other activities you enjoy, and so forth. It is very important that you do not let chronic stress and its related emotions to continue to build up inside you.

Minimizing Your Exposure to Environmental Toxins

In today's world, it is extremely important to be aware of the carcinogenic chemicals and toxins we are all in danger of being exposed to on a daily basis. This includes such chemicals and toxins found in many commercial household and garden products, cosmetics, medications, toothpaste, mouth-wash, and dental filling materials, as well as in our air, water, and food supplies. Such common items as furniture polish, car interior cleaners, and even common cleansers contain carcinogens ranging from formaldehyde to crystalline silica. While none of these products alone may present a critical carcinogenic exposure, when multiple exposures are added together, they become cumulative, stressing the body's immune system and damaging cells until, eventually, cancer sets in.

In addition, many chemicals used in cosmetics, pesticides, and other products do not require full safety testing before they are allowed to be marketed and used by millions of consumers. Therefore, it is important to gain as much information as possible about the dangerous materials to which you may be exposed, and to do all you can to avoid such chemical-laden commodities.

It is also vital that you avoid consuming food crops grown with pesticides, herbicides, and other additives, and avoid farm-raised fish and commercially raised meats and poultry, which are typically laced with antibiotics, grown hormones, and potential carcinogens. For the same reason, you should drink only pure, filtered, water and do your best to avoid areas of air pollution.

Minimize Your Exposure to Electromagnetic Fields

Our modern world is increasingly becoming one in which we are all exposed to potentially harmful radiation from the electromagnetic energy fields (EMFs) emitted from our cell phones, cell phone towers, computers, tablets, WiFi, so-called "smart meters" used by utility companies, and even our new model cars. The United States Congress' Office of Technology Assessment recommends a policy of prudent avoidance of EMFs. This means measuring electromagnetic fields in our homes and places of work and doing all we can to reduce exposure to EMFs. To measure electromagnetic radiation, you can use a gauss meter, a device that measures the amount of gauss, or magnetic flux density, occurring in the home or workspace. Gauss meters are widely available, easy to use, and can quickly help you discover sources of EMF exposure.

WiFi and cell phones are perhaps the two biggest exposures to EMFs that most people face each day. Both offer many advantages, yet a growing body of research, which is all too often ignored, continues to find that both of these technological advances pose serious potential health risks. For that reason, WiFi in schools has now been banned in parts of Canada, as well as in various European countries, while health experts now warn against placing cell phones in direct contact with one's head, carrying them in one's pockets when they are on, and sleeping beside them. I personally rarely use a cell phone, and do so primarily when traveling. When I use it, I either text or use the speaker option so that I never have to place my cell phone near my head. And when I am not using it, I always turn it off. You can do the same thing.

If, like me, you have WiFi in your home, you can do as I do an disconnect the router before going to sleep. You should also try to avoid living or working in areas that are in close proximity to power lines and electrical generating stations. Also avoid using electric blankets, electric heating pads, waterbed heaters, and similar appliances, all of which emit EMFs. And consider purchasing computer shields, which can be placed on computer screens or beneath computers to reduce exposure to electric and magnetic fields.

CONCLUSION

More than fifty years of research has established that curcumin is useful for helping to prevent and treat different types of cancer. Among its anticancer traits are curcumin's strong antioxidant and anti-inflammatory properties, and its proven ability to induce the death of cancer cells and prevent them from forming their own blood supply. Equally important, no serious adverse effects have been reported by humans taking curcumin, even at high doses.

With cancer now being the number one cause of death of people under the age of eighty-five in the United States, curcumin's anticancer properties are of growing importance. Because of the compelling body of scientific evidence supporting its effectiveness as an anticancer agent, you can understand why curcumin is recommended by a growing number of health experts as one of the most important natural compounds you can use to help protect yourself from cancer and maintain overall good health.

In the next chapter, you will learn how and why turmeric and curcumin can also help protect you against heart disease.

5

How Turmeric Can Keep Your Heart Healthy

Your heart is one of the most important organs in your body, perhaps the most important, even more so than your brain. And in today's world, it is under constant assault due to a combination of chronic stress, poor diet and nutrition, and the onslaught of environmental toxins found in our air, water, soil, and food.

Since the beginning of the twentieth century, heart disease in the United States has been our nation's number one killer. Nor is it likely to give up that position any time soon. Consider these grim statistics:

- More than 2,200 Americans die of heart disease each and every day. That's an average of one death every thirty-nine seconds.

- An average of 150,000 Americans who die of heart disease each year are younger than sixty-five years of age, while 33 percent of all deaths caused by heart disease occur before the age of seventy-five years, which is well below the average life expectancy of 77.9 years.

- Coronary heart disease causes one of every six deaths in the United States each year, while one out of every eighteen deaths is caused by stroke.

- Nearly 634,000 Americans die of heart disease each year.

- Each year, an estimated 785,000 Americans have a heart attack, and 470,000 more have a repeat attack.

- Approximately 195,000 Americans experience a silent (unnoticed or undiagnosed) first myocardial infarction each year.

- Approximately every twenty-five seconds an American will have a coronary event, and approximately every minute someone will die of one.

Once mistakenly thought to primarily affect men, approximately 50 percent of all deaths caused by heart disease in the United States each year occur among women, accounting for more than six times the number of deaths caused by breast cancer. Though mortality rates caused by heart disease have started to decline over the past decade, the overall toll continues to rise, both in terms of impaired health and financial cost. More than 1,100,000 inpatient angioplasty procedures are performed in the United States each year, along with 416,000 inpatient bypass procedures, more than 1,000,000 inpatient diagnostic cardiac catheterizations, 116,000 inpatient implantable defibrillator procedures, and 397,000 pacemaker procedures.

Annually, heart disease in the United States accounts for direct and indirect costs of more than $190.3 billion, and predictions are that these costs will increase by a minimum of 200 percent over the next twenty years. And that does not include the additional tens of billions of dollars that are spent each year to manage risk factors associated with heart disease, such as the $19 billion spent annually on statin drugs to treat elevated cholesterol levels.

Certainly there would be no reason to object to these staggering financial costs if the procedures and medications used to treat heart disease truly did their job. Unfortunately, all too often they do not. Studies show that far too common surgical procedures, such as angioplasty and bypass, are of questionable value in terms of long-term health outcomes, and can even make patients' conditions worse due to doctor error. Additional studies are also now calling into question the use of statin drugs, especially as a preventive measure for heart attack. Moreover, researchers from McMaster University in Ontario, Canada, recently discovered that nearly half of all patients who are prescribed cholesterol-lowering statin drugs get no benefit from them due to high blood levels of a protein called resistin. Resistin, which is secreted by fat tissue, causes the formation of LDL cholesterol, thus counteracting any positive effects statin drugs may have.

Although the overall incidence of death caused by heart disease is at last beginning to show signs of decline, the cost involved in treating and preventing it continues to rise at an alarming rate, and many patients continue to suffer declining quality of life issues due to the procedures and medications they receive. Surely there has to be a better way to treat and prevent our nation's number one health scourge.

While the search for such solutions continues, one of the things you can do right now to protect your heart is to add turmeric to your diet and consider supplementing with a high quality curcumin product. To understand why this is so, let's first take a closer look at the magnificent organ that your heart is and explore a bit more what causes heart disease.

MEET YOUR HEART

The human heart is the very first organ to form in the developing fetus. It begins to take shape only eighteen days after conception, and by day twenty-two it is already starting to beat and pulse. As it develops, it forms specialized muscles comprised of not just the four heart chambers (the upper left and right chambers, called the atria, and the lower left and right chambers, known as the ventricles), but also the muscle cells of the veins and arteries, as well as the tissues that make up the valves and other aspects of the heart. This complex, interrelated network is the cardiovascular system, also known as the circulatory system.

In addition to the heart itself, four main types of blood vessels make up your body's cardiovascular system: arteries, veins, capillaries, and sinusoids. All of them are shaped like hollow tubes. Healthy arteries and veins have a high degree of elasticity so that blood can flow freely through them. Combined, if all of your body's blood vessels were stretched out end to end, they would be about 60,000 miles long. That's more than twice the circumference of the earth. This astonishing fact is even more amazing when you realize that your heart moves the approximately 6 quarts (5.6 liters) of blood that are contained in the adult human body through this entire network—an average of three times every minute of your life (once every twenty seconds).

Complex as your cardiovascular system is in general, your heart is even more so. In fact, it is the most complex of all your body's organs. Though most people think of the heart simply as an organ that pumps blood, it does far more than that. It also acts like an endocrine gland, producing its own hormones, and has a rich neural tissue, comparable to the neural tissue of your brain. Perhaps this is why, throughout civilizations of the distant past, the heart was regarded as a symbol of both intelligence and intuition.

In ancient Greece, the heart was believed to be the seat of the soul, or spirit, while the ancient Chinese recognized it as the center of happiness. The Greeks were also the first to associate the heart with love. In ancient Egypt, the heart was regarded as the source of both intelligence and emotion. In fact, prior to the process of mummification, Egyptians would cut out the brain from the body and dispose of it because it was deemed unimportant, while the heart was protected so that it could guide the deceased into the afterlife.

Research has established that the heart is the greatest source of electromagnetic energy in the body. Its electrical field is sixty times greater than that of the brain, while the heart's magnetic field is 5,000 times stronger than the brain's. This cardio-electromagnetic field has been measured and extends between eight to ten feet from your body. Researchers now theorize that this field acts as a "carrier wave" of and for information, providing a global syn-chronizing signal for the entire human body.

Here are some other amazing facts about your heart:

- On average, the adult human heart only weighs between eight and ten ounces in women and men respectively, and is about the size of a fist (approximately 3.5 by 5 inches).

- Although many people believe the heart is located on the left side of their chest, in reality it is located in the center, between both lungs. Your left lung is smaller than your right lung, however, so that your heart can fit within your chest cavity.

- Your heart is almost entirely composed of muscle, and the amount of work that it performs in a single hour is enough to lift a small car weighing approximately 3,000 pounds one foot off the ground.

- The heart beats an average of 103,000 times per day every day of your life. That equates to approximately 3,600,000 times a year, and 2.5 billion times over a seventy-year-long lifespan.

- The heartbeat in women is faster than it is in men.

- The average amount of blood pumped per heartbeat when you are at rest is 2.5 ounces. Over the course of twenty-four hours that is nearly 2,000 gal-lons (approximately 20,000 pounds) of blood that your heart has moved.

- The pressure created in your heart during a single heartbeat is enough to squirt blood a distance of nearly thirty feet.

- The sound of your heartbeat is caused by closing of the valves that sepa-rate the atria from the ventricle (atrioventricular valves).

- Electrical impulses in the heart muscle (myocardium) are what causes your heart to beat.

- Laughing is very beneficial for your heart and can improve blood flow for up to forty-five minutes after you stop laughing.

- Your heart replaces your body's entire store of ATP (adenosine triphos-phate, your body's main source of energy) 8,640 times per day, or once every ten seconds.

THE REAL CAUSE OF HEART DISEASE

Contrary to popular thought, cholesterol, by itself, is not the threat to a healthy heart that most people, including physicians, continue to believe it to be. In large part, this belief in the high cholesterol model of heart disease persists because the American Heart Association and other health organizations continue to warn against high cholesterol. Yet, a growing body of research has established that cholesterol levels per se are not the problem. In fact, without cholesterol, your body simply could not function properly.

Cholesterol, particularly LDL cholesterol, becomes a threat when it has become oxidized. As this oxidation process occurs, it can result in persistent inflammation in the body, including within the arteries. Today, it is increasingly being recognized by both researchers and physicians that it is this interrelated process of oxidation and inflammation, not cholesterol, per se, that is the primary cause of heart disease. Based on this new understanding, since the 1990s, a growing number of cardiologists and other physicians have begun moving away from the high cholesterol model of heart disease, recognizing its inherently flawed premise. In place of this model, they are shifting their focus to chronic low-grade inflammation, or the "inflamed artery" model.

The theory that heart disease is caused by chronic inflammation is actually not new. In fact, it was first proposed in the nineteenth century by the physician regarded as the father of modern pathology, Dr. Rudolf Virchow. Dr. Virchow theorized that atherosclerosis, a common precursor to heart disease, was an inflammatory disease more than 150 years ago. But it was not until the late twentieth century that physicians began to seriously consider chronic inflammation's role in heart disease. Two published scientific papers, in particular, played critical roles in this shift.

The first paper was a monograph published in 1998 by the American Heart Association and edited by its president, Valentin Fuster, MD, PhD, director of the Cardiovascular Institute at Mount Sinai School of Medicine in New York City. The paper stated that 85 percent of all heart attacks and strokes were due to vulnerable plaque: a "soft" form of cholesterol, proteins, and blood cells that builds up within the arterial wall. The findings of the monograph were widely reported in both conventional medical journals and the mainstream media and debunked the belief that heart disease is primarily due to hard arterial plaque that obstructs the artery (the high cholesterol/ blocked artery model). Given the fact that Dr. Fuster is the only cardiologist to receive four major research awards from the world's top four cardiovascular organizations (the AHA, the American College of Cardiology, the European Society of Cardiology, and the InterAmerican Society of Cardiology), the monograph proved quite influential.

As the monograph explained, vulnerable plaque primarily consists of soft cholesterol and clotting proteins that are different than the type of obstructing plaque common in atherosclerosis, and which is contained by a fibrous cap that is thinner and weaker than obstructing plaque and more easily ruptured. The body reacts to vulnerable plaque in much the same way that it deals with infection, releasing blood cells to attack and inflame the fibrous cap. This attack, and the inflammation that results from it, can cause the cap to break, spilling the powerful coagulants found in its interior into the bloodstream, where they can form large and lethal clots.

Cardiologists now believe that vulnerable plaque explains why some people with little or no blockages in their arteries can still have heart attacks, while others with almost completely blocked arteries may never experience any symptoms of heart disease. In the "inflamed artery" model of heart disease, plaque in the arteries is regarded as a mechanism the body uses to repair damage in the arterial walls. In response to such tears, the body releases various substances into the bloodstream to adhere, or stick, to the site of the tears. There, these substances attract a special class of cells called platelets, which are responsible for clotting, and together they combine to form the protective fibrous cap. It is the integrity of the cap itself that determines the stability of the plaque.

It is now recognized that oxidized cholesterol, as well as chronic infection, can trigger the formation of vulnerable plaque, setting in motion a vicious cycle, since the inflammation response is one of the ways your body deals with both oxidized cholesterol and infections. When vulnerable plaque comes in contact with oxidized cholesterol or infections, the body, in its attempt to prevent the further spread of these substances, causes the blood passing through the infected area to become hyper-coagulable and viscous. A clot may also form, impeding blood flow. Left untreated, this process can eventually result in heart disease and possibly death.

In 2002, another major scientific paper expanded the findings of the Fuster monograph, and truly laid the cornerstone for the emerging chronic inflammation/"inflamed artery" model of heart disease. Written by lead author Dr. Peter Libby, chief of cardiovascular medicine at the Brigham and Women's Hospital in Boston, MA, and director of the D.W. Reynolds Cardiovascular Clinical Research Center at Harvard University, the paper published in the prestigious medical journal *Circulation*. The paper, entitled *Inflammation and Atherosclerosis*, proved to be a seminal article that has subsequently been cited in no less than 9,500 other scientific papers.

As Dr. Libby pointed out, atherosclerosis occurs when various white blood cells that act as the first line of defense against infectious agents take hold and become active in arterial tissue. At the onset of this process, small particles of LDL cholesterol begin to accumulate within the artery wall. As they do so, they start to be altered chemically. Then the modified LDL cholesterol triggers the artery's endothelial cells to release molecules that latch on to immune cells in the blood (primarily monocytes and T-cells). At the same time, the endothelial cells secrete chemicals called *chemokines* that entice the snared immune cells into the innermost layer of the artery's membrane structure.

Once inside this membrane structure, monocyte immune cells transform into macrophages that seek out and ingest the modified LDL cholesterol. As they do so, the macrophages fill up with fatty droplets until they are so laden with fat that they become what are known as foam cells. Meanwhile, T-cells also ensnared within the membrane start to form the earliest stages of plaque. Plaque buildup and growth is further promoted by other inflammatory molecules, triggering the formation of the fibrous cap that is characteristic of vulnerable plaque. This cap increases the size of the plaque while also walling it off from the blood. However, over time, other inflammatory substances secreted by the foam cells weaken the cap and can cause it to rupture. Should such a rupture occur, dangerous blood clots can form, ultimately leading to heart attack or stroke.

HOW TURMERIC AND CURCUMIN CAN PROTECT YOUR HEART

It's long been established that diets rich in antioxidant foods can prevent free radical damage, chronic inflammation, and the oxidation process. Because of this, such diets have also long been recommended for people who have or who are at risk of developing heart disease. Turmeric also acts as a potent antioxidant, as does curcumin.

In Chapter 2, you learned about the ability of both turmeric and curcumin to prevent and help reverse chronic inflammation. Given the primary role chronic inflammation plays in triggering and worsening heart disease, you can understand why a growing body of research has led to more and more doctors and other health experts recommending turmeric and curcumin supplements to their patients in order to improve the health of their hearts and help protect against heart disease. In addition, due to the B vitamins turmeric contains, adding it as spice to your diet can also provide another important benefit for your heart and cardiovascular system. That's because B vitamins help regulate and prevent elevated levels of homocysteine.

Homocysteine is a naturally-occurring amino acid in the body, and is also obtained by eating protein-rich foods, especially meat. High levels of homocysteine in the body is today considered to be a risk factor for heart disease. The reason for this is because elevated homocysteine levels have been found to increase the likelihood of atherosclerosis (hardening of the arteries), as well as unhealthy blood clots, which can lead to stroke.

The standard American diet is deficient in B vitamins, as well as many of the other nutrients turmeric contains (see Chapter 1). Making turmeric a part of your diet can help to rectify this problem, and also help keep your body's homocysteine levels under control.

But turmeric's general anti inflammation, anti oxidation, and homocyc teine-lowering properties are only three of the many important heart-healthy benefits the spice, along with curcumin, provide. These other benefits include:

- aiding in the transport of calcium out of heart muscle cells.

- increasing healthy HDL cholesterol levels while lowering so-called "bad" LDL cholesterol levels.

- protecting against an enlarged heart (cardiac hypertrophy).

- protecting against high blood pressure (hypertension).

- reducing plaque buildup in the arteries and protecting against athero-sclerosis (hardening of the arteries).

Let's examine how and why turmeric and curcumin provide each of these benefits in turn.

Improved Cholesterol Levels

As you learned earlier in this chapter, although cholesterol of itself is not a risk factor for heart disease, a healthy ratio of HDL to LDL cholesterol remains important for maintaining the health of your heart. A healthy total cholesterol count (the sum of HDL and LDL levels when they are combined together) is also important. A number of human clinical trials have confirmed that turmeric and curcumin provide benefits for each of this category. This is particularly true of curcumin.

In one such study, for example, daily supplementation with 500 mg of curcumin increased HDL levels by 29 percent after only seven days. The study involved ten healthy men and women. In the same study, the participants' total cholesterol levels decreased by 12 percent. More importantly, according to the researchers who oversaw this study, the participants also experienced a "33 percent decrease in serum lipid peroxidases." Lipid peroxidation is a process of oxidation caused by free radicals "stealing" electrons from the lip-ids (fats) in cell membranes. This, in turn, results in cellular damage, which, when left unchecked, can cause a chain reaction of ongoing free radical damage, as well as inflammation and oxidation of cholesterol. Remember, it is when cholesterol becomes inflamed and oxidized that it truly poses a danger to your heart.

In another study, which involved seventy-five patients suffering from acute coronary syndrome, daily supplementation with curcumin was also found to improve cholesterol levels. The study was a randomized, double-blind clinical trial conducted over a period of one year and involved both men and women, all of whom had similar lab readings with regard to their cholesterol levels (HDL, LDL, and total cholesterol), triglycerides, blood glucose levels, and other parameters. The participants were divided into four groups, with three of the groups given a different dose of curcumin three times each day, with the fourth group serving as a control. The doses ranged from low, to moderate, to high (15, 30, and 60 mg of curcumin three times a day). By the study's end, the researchers found that all three curcumin groups had achieved lower LDL and total cholesterol scores, as well as improved (raised) HDL scores.

More recently, a meta-analysis of seven other studies involving a total of 649 patients with risk factors for cardiovascular disease found that both turmeric and curcumin "significantly reduced" the patients' LDL cholesterol and triglcyerides readings, and also lowered their blood lipid levels, compared to patients in the studies' respective control groups.

Protecting Against Atherosclerosis

Atherosclerosis, or hardening of the arteries, is a chronic, progressive disease caused by inflammation and oxidation within the arterial linings, or walls, as well as the aorta (the main trunk or the artery system that transports blood from the left side of the heart to the arteries of all of the body's limbs and organs, except the lungs). As it takes hold, lesions form on these walls or within the aorta, causing them to harden and narrow. This situation is made worse by the platelets that migrate and clump around the lesion sites, coupled with peroxidation of fats within the arteries.

Both animal and human studies have demonstrated turmeric's and curcumin's ability to help prevent and reverse atherosclerosis. One of the primary reasons why they are able to do so lies in their proven ability to prevent and reverse inflammatory and oxidative damage to cholesterol, especially LDL cholesterol. Studies have also shown that curcumin is able to reduce atherosclerotic lesions in both the arteries and aorta. Additional research indicates that curcumin can also help prevent platelets from clumping within the arteries.

Protecting Against High Blood Pressure

High blood pressure, or hypertension, is a serious condition that can lead to other health problems, including heart attack and stroke. According to the American Heart Association, approximately one-third of all American adults have high blood pressure, including many people in their early twenties. Another third of all Americans suffer from pre-hypertension, meaning their blood pressure levels are higher than normal.

In addition, all too often high blood pressure goes undiagnosed. Over 20 percent of people with high blood pressure are not aware of their condition. For this reason, high blood pressure is often referred to as "the silent killer" because the damage it can cause within the body can go undetected until it is too late to prevent heart attack, stroke, and other conditions. Although high blood pressure is not a disease, per se, it is a valuable marker for heart disease, and therefore it is important that it be monitored.

Although the effects of turmeric and curcumin on high blood pressure have not been studied extensively, preliminary research conducted on animals has demonstrated that curcumin in particular can help protect against hypertension in a number of important ways. First and foremost, curcumin has been found to directly suppress elevated blood pressure levels. Of equal importance, it is also capable of causing arteries to relax by inducing vasodilation. It does this by promoting the release of nitric oxide (NO) in arteries due to its antioxidant properties. NO is known to help counteract high blood pressure and enhance overall cardiovascular function. Finally, in a study with humans suffering from a type of kidney disease called lupus nephritis, curcumin supplements were found to decrease their systolic blood pressure levels. (Systolic blood pressure is the pressure in the artery when the heart pumps. It typically measures higher than diastolic blood pressure, which is the pressure in the artery when the heart relaxes. Blood pressure readings of 120 (systolic)/80 (diastolic) mmHg are considered normal.)

Protecting Against An Enlarged Heart

When the heart is under stress it can become enlarged, with the enlargement primarily occurring in the myocardium, the middle muscular layer of the heart wall. This condition is known as *cardiac hypertrophy*, which, over time, can lead to heart failure and death. During the onset and progression of cardiac hypertrophy, the expression of various genes in the heart become altered due to the influence of a specific type of enzymes called *histone acetyltransferases*, or HATs.

HATs, because of the way they interact with histone proteins, are capable of turning genes in the heart on or off. In the case of cardiac hypertrophy, a particular HAT known as p300-HAT plays a significant role because it can increase the expression of genes that, in turn, cause the myocardium to enlarge.

Animal studies have shown that curcumin inhibits the action of p300-HAT and suppresses the hypertrophic responses that p300-HAT can trigger in the cells of the myocardium. In addition, studies have also found that these properties of curcumin were capable of preventing heart failure in animals in which cardiac hypertrophy had previously been induced.

Moving Calcium Out of Heart Muscle Cells

While calcium is certainly an important mineral that is necessary for good health, an excess of calcium in the body, particular inside of the cells, can cause a variety of serious problems, including atherosclerosis and other risk factors for heart disease. Because of this, many nutritionally oriented cardiologists and other physicians are no longer recommending calcium supplements for their patients, including women, emphasizing instead that we obtain the mineral from food, especially calcium-rich green vegetables, rather than milk and dairy products.

All the cells in your body, including the cells in your heart, are involved in a delicate balance that interchanges ions of calcium and sodium with magnesium and potassium ions. For the most part, both calcium and sodium belong outside of the cell wall, while magnesium and potassium belong inside of cells. All four of these mineral ions pass in and out of the cells, however, and are balanced by a cellular mechanism known as the *sodium-potassium pump.* In the heart, this "pump" plays an important role in maintaining the chemical reactions that are necessary for the heart's muscle fibers to properly band together and contract. The sodium-potassium pump allows calcium ions inside heart fibers when they contract, and then ushers them out again so that magnesium can reenter and initiate the relaxation phase.

Excess calcium levels in the body can disrupt this balance, leading to too many calcium ions inside heart cells known as *cardiomyocites.* When this happens, the heart is forced to contract more forcefully. This, in turn, increases blood pressure levels and can lead to chronic hypertension, and can also cause angina. To counteract these negative effects, cardiologists often prescribe calcium channel-blocking drugs. As with most heart medications and other drugs, they carry the risk of serious side effects. Fortunately, there is a better solution.

Research has shown that both turmeric and curcumin improve the transport of calcium into and out of heart cells the way that nature intended. According to researchers, this is due to their positive effects on a compound

Curcumin Is as Effective as Aerobic Exercise in Protecting Against Heart Disease

In addition to all of the above benefits, researchers in Japan documented multiple ways in which curcumin can provide the same overall cardiovascular benefits as those that are provided from regular moderate aerobic exercise. Aerobic exercise has, for many years, been recommended as an important step to maintaining good cardiovascular health, making these findings especially noteworthy for people who, because of their overall health status, are unable to exercise.

The Japanese researchers conducted three clinical trials, all of which involved postmenopausal women, an age group that has a higher risk for heart disease. The studies were randomized, double-blind, and placebo-controlled, and were conducted by researchers at Japan's University of Tsukuba. The studies' results demonstrated that daily supplementation with curcumin improved endothelial (artery) function, as well as other heart disease-related risk factors to the same degree that moderate aerobic exercise does. As the researchers of one of the studies wrote, "[R]egular ingestion of curcumin could be a preventive measure against cardiovascular disease in postmenopausal women. Furthermore, our results suggest that curcumin may be a potential alternative . . . for patients who are unable to exercise."

The first of the studies compared the effects of moderate aerobic exercise and curcumin on blood flow. In the study, thirty-two postmenopausal women were randomly assigned to one of three groups for an eight-week trial period. The first group acted as the control, or placebo group, the second received curcumin supplements once each day, and the third engaged in moderate aerobic exercise training.

The women's vascular health was assessed before and after the study using a test that measures "flow-mediated dilation," or FMD. FMD scores can help predict a person's risk for developing heart disease. In fact, recent studies have found that every 1 percent drop in FMD increases the risk of heart disease by 12 percent.

The women in both the aerobic exercise and curcumin groups increased their FMD scores by 1.5 percent by the study's conclusion, while there were changes in the control group during that same period.

The second study examined curcumin's effects on artery response compared to moderate aerobic exercise. This study also involved thirty-two postmenopausal women and was conducted over an eight-week period. The women were randomly assigned to one of four groups, with the first group serving as the control group. They were given placebo pills. The women in the second group received a curcumin supplement once a day. The third group of women engaged in moderate aerobic exercise and received the same placebo pills as the women in the first group. The fourth group both engaged in moderate aerobic exercise and also received a daily curcumin supplement.

The aim of this study was to measure the effects of curcumin, moderate exercise, and a combination of the two on what is known as their *arterial compliance* (AC). AC is another significant indicator of a person's overall artery (vascular) health. It refers to the change in a person's blood volume in response to changes in blood pressure levels. Like FMD scores, AC scores can also predict the risk for heart disease. The women's AC scores were measured before and at the end of the clinical study period.

In all but the control group, the AC scores improved by the study's completion, whereas the control group's scores remained the same. The results of the study also demonstrated those who received curcumin each day had the same level of improvement in their scores as did the women who engaged in daily moderate aerobic exercise. As you might expect, the AC scores in the women who both engaged in daily exercise and received curcumin supplements were found to have the greatest improvement in their AC scores

According to the researchers who conducted this study, curcumin's ability to improve AC scores is likely due to the effect it has on the genes that regulate proteins in the immune system that trigger both inflammation and oxidation, especially a protein known as tumor necrosis factor-alpha (TNF-alpha). The researchers wrote, "Curcumin exerts anti-inflammatory and anti-oxidative effects by inhibiting tumor necrosis factor-alpha (TNF-alpha) . . . [h]owever, TNF-alpha levels were not assessed in this study. . . . Further studies are warranted to clarify the mechanism underlying the effect of curcumin on endothelial [blood vessel] function."

In the third clinical trial, which also was conducted over an eight-week period, forty-five postmenopausal women were randomly assigned to four groups. As in the second study, they consisted of a control group that received placebo pills, a group that received a daily curcumin supplement, a group that engaged in moderate aerobic exercise, and a final group in which curcumin and exercise were combined.

The purpose of this study was to examine the effects of curcumin and moderate aerobic exercise, individually and when combined, have on the women's blood pumping pressure, specifically what is known as left ventricular (LV) afterload. LV afterload refers to the stress that is placed on the heart's left ventricle as it ejects blood from the heart to the rest of the body. A primary factor for determining LV afterload is the aortic and pulmonary pressure the left ventricular muscle needs to overcome in order to eject blood from the heart. The higher the degree of aortic/pulmonary pressure there is, the higher the LV afterload will be as well. As the LV afterload level increases the volume of the blood being pumped by the heart decreases, leading to a greater risk for heart disease. For most people, LV afterload levels increase as they age.

Before and after this study, the LV afterload levels of the women in all four groups was determined by measuring their aortic and brachial systolic blood pressure levels, as well as what is known as their heart-rate corrected aortic augmentation index (AIx). AIx is a measurement that helps physicians determine how efficiently their patients arteries are functioning.

As in the other two studies, the women in the control group showed no improvements in these three measurements, whereas all the women in the remaining three groups did. Once again, the curcumin and moderate exercise groups showed equals levels of improvement, but the most significant improvements occurred in the women who both exercised and received a daily curcumin supplement. In this group, all three measurements dropped most significantly, leading the researchers of this study to write, "These findings suggest that regular endurance exercise combined with daily curcumin ingestion may reduce LV after load to a greater extent than monotherapy [single therapy] with either intervention alone in postmenopausal women."

known as *plasma membrane calcium ATPase* (PMCA). PMCA is a type of transport protein that serves to regulate the amount of calcium inside of cells, including heart cells, as well as removing calcium from cells. Scientists have discovered that turmeric and especially curcumin enhance PMCA function and, as a result, may even be able to correct defective calcium homeostasis within the muscles of the heart itself.

OTHER TIPS FOR KEEPING YOUR HEART HEALTHY

Adding turmeric to your diet and taking a curcumin supplement are, of course, hardly the only things you need to do to keep your heart healthy. Although a full discussion on heart health is beyond the scope of this book, here are some other important tips that can help you protect your heart.

Diet

The food choices you make each day are one of the most important factors that determine how healthy you will be. For better heart and overall health, the best diet is one that is low in unhealthy fats (both trans-fats as well as an excessive intake of omega-6 fatty acids, which cause inflammation in the body), low in sugar and simple carbohydrates, and rich in unprocessed, ideally organic, foods, including lean organ meats, fish, and plenty of fiber-rich fresh fruits and vegetables. Whole grains and legumes are also healthy, although research continues to find that even healthy carbohydrates should only be eaten in moderation. Also be sure to drink plenty of pure, filtered water throughout the day, as well as fresh coconut milk or water if it is available. And for cooking and baking purposes, use extra virgin coconut oil.

Exercise

Regular exercise is essential. However, contrary to popular opinion, exercise does not have to be intense or prolonged in order for you to benefit from it. In fact, prolonged periods of intense exercise has now been found to increase inflammation levels in the body. For best results, choose a type of exercise or physical activity you enjoy, such as a regular, daily twenty minute walk, bicycling, or swimming.

Lifestyle

Adopting a healthy lifestyle is also vitally important. This means not smoking and avoiding secondhand smoke, and limiting your intake of caffeine and alcoholic drinks (especially hard alcohol; one or two glasses of beer or red wine each day is not only permissible but also good for your heart). Losing weight, if you need to do so, is also important.

Overall, a healthy lifestyle is one in which you avoid the choices above and replace them with heart-healthy meals and regular physical activity, along with engaging in other activities you enjoy, such as a favorite hobby, which can promote relaxation and increase happiness. Also make it a point to spend quality time with your family and friends. Such healthy lifestyles choices will also help you to better cope with stress, which is also vitally important, given how closely associated chronic stress is with heart disease.

CONCLUSION

As this chapter makes clear, despite all of the marvelous advances that have been made to detect and treat it, heart disease continues to be our nation's number one killer. However, by understanding the major risk factors that cause heart disease, it is my hope that you now understand there is much you can do on your own to protect yourself and your loved ones from experiencing heart attack, stroke, or other types of heart disease. I hope you also now understand how and why turmeric and curcumin can also go a long way towards maintaining a healthy heart.

In the next chapter, you will discover the benefits turmeric and curcumin can provide in regard to your digestion and ability to defend against gastro-intestinal conditions.

6

Turmeric Improves Digestion & Protects Against Gastrointestinal Conditions

Good digestion and an optimally functioning gastrointestinal (GI) tract—your gut—are both vitally important to your overall health. Hippocrates, the "Father of Western Medicine," is famous for his saying, "Let food by thy medicine, and medicine thy food." He taught more than 2,500 years ago that most illness begins because of disturbances in the GI tract. Yet, today poor digestion and gastrointestinal problems are among the most common health complaints experienced by Americans. This fact alone goes a long way towards explaining why, as a nation, the United States is beset with such a widespread incidence of chronic disease conditions.

At the same time, researchers continue to confirm what Hippocrates pointed out so long ago. Based on their research, we now have scientific proof that the effects of poor digestion and gastrointestinal problems are not limited to the GI tract alone. Impaired functioning of the GI tract negatively affects your body's immune system, causing or exacerbating a wide range of immune deficiency-related diseases, including cancer.

More recently, scientists have discovered that poor gastrointestinal health plays a significant role in poor brain health. It can also affect memory and cognitive function, and is a major cause of neurological conditions, including Alzheimer's disease, dementia, and Parkinson's disease. In addition, impaired GI function contributes to various mental health issues, such as anxiety and depression, and is one of the main causes of chronic fatigue. GI problems can also interfere with your ability to achieve deep, restful sleep.

Based on these facts, you can see why healthy digestion and achieving and maintaining good gastrointestinal tract functioning is so important to your overall health. In this chapter, you are going to learn how turmeric and curcumin can help you to do so. First, though, let's take a quick look at what your gastrointestinal tract actually is and what it does.

MEET YOUR GASTROINTESTINAL TRACT

The gastrointestinal tract begins at the mouth and ends at the anus. In essence, it is a hollow tube known as the alimentary canal, and in adults ranges in length from 25 to 32 feet, depending on a person's height. It consists of the mouth, larynx, pharynx, esophagus, stomach, small intestine (comprised of three sections: the duodenum, jejunum, and illeum), large intestine (comprised of the cecum, ascending colon, transverse colon, and descending colon), rectum, and anus. In addition, the GI tract is supported by the gallbladder, liver, and pancreas, all of which play vital roles in the process of digestion.

The GI tract performs two equally important functions. First, it digests the foods you consume and makes the vital nutrients and other compounds these foods contain available to the rest of the body. Then it assembles wastes and other food byproducts and eliminates them through defecation.

Digestion begins in the mouth when we chew our food. As we do so, our salivary glands release enzymes that begin the process of breaking down food and separating out the nutrients it contains. Then, as food is swallowed, this process is further carried out in the stomach, where hydrochloric acid (HCl), which is essential for the proper digestion of protein, and pepsin, an enzyme that also helps break down proteins, are secreted. While in the stomach, food becomes liquefied as it interacts with HCl and pepsin, and then moves onto the small intestine. There it interacts with additional enzymes that are secreted by the pancreas. These enzymes include protease, which further digests proteins; amylase, which digests carbohydrates; and lipase, which digests fats.

It is in the small intestine that the liver and gallbladder also contribute to the process of digestion. Both of these organs secrete bile, which stimulates the small intestine and is essential for the proper absorption of fats and the fat soluble vitamins A, D, E, and K contained in food. The liver also detoxifies food and metabolizes cholesterol. Most of the absorption of the nutrients food contains occurs here, in the small intestine. Water, electrolytes, and remaining food products are absorbed in the large intestine. What is left over (toxins, waste byproducts, and undigested food particles) then passes out of the large intestine to be eliminated from the body.

Healthy intestinal flora, or bacteria, play a primary role in helping maintain the health of the GI tract and ensuring proper digestion and elimination. In addition, they also play important roles in hormone regulation, the GI tract's production of certain vitamins, such as B vitamins, and targeting toxins. Moreover, research has now found that healthy bacterial balance in the GI tract is important for a person's overall mental and emotional health.

Scientists have determined that there are over 500 different species of healthy bacteria that reside in the GI tract. All told, there are ten times as many of these bacteria in your GI tract than the total number of your body's cells.

Another important feature of the GI tract is the vast network of lymph channels that are contained within the walls of the small intestine. This network transports lymph to the rest of the body. Lymph is a clear fluid that contains various cells that are essential for the formation of antibodies used by the body to fight off infection. It is this large reservoir of lymph channels in the small intestine that is one of the reasons why your GI tract, when healthy, is so vital to the health of your body's immune system.

The gastrointestinal tract also houses the enteric nervous system (ENS), which scientists have dubbed the body's "second brain." The ENS is located in the linings of the esophagus, stomach, small intestine, and colon, and is one of the main divisions within your body's overall nervous system. It is made up of an array of neurons, which contain neurotransmitter proteins that govern the functioning of the GI tract. These neurotransmitter proteins are produced by cells identical to those found in the brain. This complex neuronal circuitry in the gut enables the GI, or second brain, to act independently, remember, and produce "gut feelings," leading credence to the adage about "trusting your gut." Additionally, the ENS is also home to over 90 percent of your body's supply of serotonin and approximately 50 percent of its dopamine supply. These two neurotransmitters have played a large role in the recent research into the interplay between what scientists now refer to as the *gut-brain axis.*

Although the ENS normally communicates with your body's central nervous system (CNS) via nerve signals sent along the pathways of the parasympathetic and sympathetic nervous systems, research has proven that it is also capable of acting autonomously (on its own). For example, animal studies have shown that when the vagus nerve, a primary pathway of the parasympathetic nervous system, is severed, the ENS is still capable of functioning properly. In addition, other animal studies have found that the various classes of neurons within the ENS enable it to properly oversee the secretion of enzymes and regulate mechanical and chemical conditions within the GI tract without input from the CNS. The ENS is also able to control peristalsis, the contraction and relaxation of the GI tract's smooth muscle tissues that move food along the alimentary canal, without input from the central nervous system.

Recent research has also found that healthy gut bacteria can positively influence the gut-brain axis. Conversely, a buildup of unhealthy gut bacteria, such as *Candida albicans*, which, when it becomes unchecked, causes systemic yeast overgrowth, or candidiasis, can disrupt the proper functioning of the gut-brain access. Unhealthy gut bacteria can also result in intestinal hyper-permeability, which is more commonly known as "leaky gut syndrome." Studies demonstrate that people who suffer from leaky gut syndrome are more likely than others to also suffer from autoimmune diseases and mental health issues such as depression and anxiety, as well as abdominal pain, bloating after meals, acid reflux, flatulence, and less obvious gut-related conditions such as headache, fatigue, and joint pain.

The buildup of unhealthy bacteria, leaky gut syndrome, poor digestion, and other gastrointestinal conditions all have one thing in common: chronic inflammation of the GI tract. Research conducted at John Hopkins Center for Neurogastroenterology and other research centers has found that, in the presence of inflammation, the ENS signals the central nervous system in ways that can cause the CNS to trigger anxiety, depression, or other negative changes in mood. Inflammation in the gut can also impair the brain's cognitive function, memory, and thinking skills, and plays a role in the development and progression of various neurological conditions, including Parkinson's disease, Alzheimer's disease, and dementia.

Given the ability of both turmeric and curcumin to prevent and reverse chronic inflammation, you can understand why both of these substances can benefit the health of your GI tract and also help relieve a variety of gastrointestinal conditions. Let's take a closer look at how and why they can do so.

HOW AND WHY TURMERIC AND CURCUMIN CAN IMPROVE THE HEALTH OF YOUR GI TRACT

In addition to the anti-inflammatory and antioxidant benefits that they provide, both turmeric and curcumin offer a number of other important benefits that aid digestion and can help relieve various gastrointestinal complaints. These include:

- enhancing both liver and pancreas function.

- improving overall stomach function.

- increasing the activity of digestive enzymes.

- preventing and helping reverse food poisoning caused by bacterial toxins or intestinal parasites.

- preventing and relieving acid reflux and heartburn.

- preventing and relieving both localized and systemic abdominal pain caused by gastrointestinal disorders.

- regulating peristalsis (contraction of the GI tract's smooth muscles) to prevent and reduce the incidence of constipation and diarrhea.

- relieving flatulence and inhibiting the formation of gas in the GI tract caused by bacterial toxins.

- relieving nausea caused by food poisoning.

- stimulating bile production in both the gallbladder and liver.

In India and other Asian countries where Ayurvedic medicine is practiced, turmeric has, for centuries, been recommended as an aid to digestion, which is one of the reasons why it is so often used as a spice to flavor traditional meals in those regions. Now that researchers have determined the positive effects turmeric has for stimulating bile and increasing digestive enzyme activity, the wisdom of this Ayurvedic recommendation has been confirmed. Because of this, in 1999, the World Health Organization recommended turmeric as a treatment for a number of gastrointestinal conditions, including acid reflux, flatulence, and indigestion in accordance with Ayurvedic precepts. So, if you wish to improve your own digestion, one of the simplest and most effective steps you can take is to add turmeric as a spice to your meals. You can also accompany your meals with a cup of turmeric tea.

In addition to research confirming that turmeric and curcumin can improve digestion, scientists have also discovered that both turmeric and curcumin can help relieve the symptoms of a number of gastrointestinal disorders. These include bloating and flatulence, colitis, Crohn's disease, food poisoning, gallstones, hemorrhoids, irritable bowel syndrome (IBS), liver and pancreas problems, and ulcers.

Bloating and Flatulence

Both bloating and flatulence (gas) are caused by the fermentation or partial digestion of foods, and also by bacterial toxins within the GI tract. As gas (flatus) in the GI tract builds up, stomach bloat can be a common result. Other symptoms include abdominal pain and chest pain, which can range from mild to severe. Severe chest pain caused by intestinal gas buildup can sometimes be mistaken for symptoms of a heart attack.

Turmeric and curcumin can help prevent and alleviate both bloating and flatulence in a number of ways. First, they can help your body more efficiently and fully digest the foods you eat by enhancing the ability of the digestive enzymes your body produces. Without an adequate supply of such enzymes, proper food digestion cannot occur. Second, as mentioned above, both turmeric and curcumin also stimulate the production of bile by the gallbladder and liver, further aiding in digestion, especially the digestion of fats.

Of equal importance, turmeric and curcumin have been shown by researchers to stop the formation of gas caused by bacterial toxins within the GI tract. Both compounds have also been shown to protect and help destroy various gastrointestinal parasites, including *Giardia* and *Cryptosporidium*, two types parasites that are found in our nation's municipal water supplies far more often than most people know.

Colitis and Crohn's Disease

Colitis (also known as ulcerative colitis) and Crohn's disease are both forms of inflammatory bowel disease (IBD). Both conditions are chronic and caused by inflammation resulting from an overactive immune response, meaning that they are both autoimmune disorders. These diseases share many of the same symptoms, which include abdominal pain and cramping, diarrhea, blood in the stool, nausea, and an abnormally increased need to evacuate the bowels.

The primary difference between the two conditions lies in where they occur within the GI tract. Colitis occurs only in the colon and rectum, whereas Crohn's disease can occur anywhere within the GI tract. In addition, unlike colitis, Crohn's disease can sometimes affect the kidneys and liver and, in some cases, even the blood, eyes, and skin. Both conditions can also significantly increase the risk of colon cancer and cancer of the rectum.

Recent population, hospital, and clinical studies from around the world have found that in northern Europe and North America, Crohn's disease is now more common than colitis is, while in eastern European countries and other undeveloped countries in Asia and elsewhere, colitis occurs more often. In addition, around the world today there is an increasing prevalence of both these conditions in men. This is a marked change from the past, when Crohn's disease was 30-percent more prevalent in women.

Researchers and physicians have yet to determine the definitive cause of colitis and Crohn's disease, but they do know that it is at least in part due to the body's immune system excessively reacting to the presence of microbes, especially bacteria, in the GI tract, including ones that, under normal conditions, would be perceived by the immune system as being benign (harmless). As this process occurs, the intestinal lining becomes more permeable, resulting in leaky gut syndrome, which, in turn, causes too much exposure and contact between the microbes and the immune system.

In addition to the overreactive immune response that is involved in both of these IBD conditions, researchers have also found that problems with the smallest blood vessels in the intestines can also cause or exacerbate IBD. These problems are caused by overstimulation of these blood vessels, causing them to abnormally grow, meaning their growth becomes unchecked. As explained in previous chapters, this unimpeded growth is known as angiogenesis, and is one of the ways that cancer tumor cells spread and thrive in the body.

Conventional medical treatment of IBD typically involves the use of systemic anti-inflammatory drugs, such as sulfasalazine and corticosteroids, anti-inflammatory suppositories, and drugs that suppress immune system functioning. In some cases, antibiotic drugs may also be prescribed, although their effectiveness for treating Crohn's disease is negligible. As is the case with the vast majority of other pharmaceutical drugs in general, the drugs used to treat IBD carry the risk for potentially serious side effects. Among them are diarrhea, liver damage, an increased risk of glaucoma, osteoporosis, and an increased risk of cancer and infectious diseases, including tuberculosis. Fortunately, turmeric and curcumin are safer alternatives.

Both animal and human clinical studies have shown that curcumin and other compounds in turmeric can safely and effectively relieve the abdominal pain and inflammation associated with IBD. Animal studies have also shown that curcumin is as effective as the drug sulfasalazine for treating IBD-related damage in the colon. Numerous other studies have shown that there are virtually no negative side effects in humans when using turmeric or its curcumin extracts to treat IBD and other GI tract conditions. In addition, research also confirms that using curcumin and other turmeric extracts, rather than systemic steroid drugs, limits suppression of the inflammatory immune system response to the intestines, thus avoiding the serious side effects that can occur from suppressing the immune system in the entire body.

Both turmeric and curcumin can help prevent and treat IBD in a number of important ways. First, clinical studies have demonstrated that they can not only prevent and block chronic inflammation in the body, they can also prevent abnormal angiogenesis in the intestines. In addition, turmeric and curcumin have been shown to be effective for regulating the body's immune response. They do so in a number of ways, including blocking pro-inflammatory proteins that trigger various helper T-cells in the immune system known to cause or exacerbate IBD, suppressing over-activation of immune system mast cells, checking the spread of lymphocytes, and preventing dentritic cells from further stimulating an already overactive immune system.

Turmeric and curcumin also provide antioxidant protection within the GI tract, thus preventing and helping to reverse free radical damage that is also a component of IBD. Finally, turmeric and curcumin have been shown to inhibit the pro-inflammatory activity of a protein complex known as NF-κB, a primary activator of inflammation in the immune system that is also known to trigger genes to produce various other inflammatory substances, including COX-2 enzymes. The reduction of COX-2 enzymes in the GI tract also significantly reduces the risk of cancer associated with IBD.

Various human studies have been conducted on the use of turmeric and curcumin as treatments for IBD, providing scientific evidence that both turmeric and curcumin are indeed effective for preventing and alleviating colitis and Crohn's disease. In addition, researchers have also shown that turmeric and curcumin are safe and effective natural treatments for keeping IBD conditions in remission once they are resolved. For example, results from one pilot clinical study of five Crohn's disease patients and another six-month placebo-controlled clinical trial of eighty-nine patients with ulcerative colitis both demonstrated that curcumin taken as a supplement not only significantly relieved the participants' symptoms, but also reduced the rate of relapse by nearly 400 percent compared to the placebo group.

Additional research has also shown that curcumin taken as an oral supplement can improve the effectiveness of pharmaceutical drugs used to treat IBD. In one double-blind study, for instance, patients were randomly selected to take the anti-inflammatory drug mesalamine with either curcumin or with a placebo. The patients who took curcumin along with mesalamine experienced greater rates of remission compared to patients who received a placebo.

Researchers have also determined, however, that the amount of curcumin taken each day is a critical factor in regard to its effectiveness. A number of studies have found that a daily dose of 2,000 to 3,000 mg of curcumin is much more effective in achieving and maintaining remission of IBD symptoms than a typical dose of 450 mg. This lower amount has also been shown to not be enough to achieve remission in the first place.

Food Poisoning

Food poisoning is caused by eating contaminated food or drinking contaminated water. The primary sources of contamination are bacterial and viral toxins or parasites. Symptoms of food poisoning include abdominal pain, diarrhea, nausea, vomiting, and overall weakness and fatigue. Turmeric and curcumin protect and alleviate symptoms of food poisoning for the same reason that they also help prevent and relieve bloating and flatulence. As mentioned previously, both turmeric and curcumin are effective in neutralizing bacterial and other microbial toxins, and in protecting against parasite infection.

Gallstones

Gallstones are hardened deposits that form inside the gallbladder and are composed of cholesterol, bile, lecithin, and other substances. Gallstones are the most common type of gallbladder problem, and are also the leading cause of surgery for gastrointestinal conditions, typically resulting in the surgical removal of the gallbladder. Gallstones are far more common in women, striking them four times as frequently as they do men.

In many cases, people with gallstones remain unaware that they have them because the stones cause no obvious symptoms. In other cases, the symptoms can be painful. Pain occurs in the right side of the abdomen, where the gallbladder is located, and may also present as pain in the right shoulder. Sometimes right-sided shoulder pain may occur by itself. Wherever the pain occurs, it is generally constant and can increase over time. Other symptoms of gallstones include nausea, heartburn, flatulence, belching, and, in some cases, vomiting, especially after eating meals that are high in fat. Large gallstones can block the gallbladder's bile ducts. Such cases often result in the removal of the gallbladder.

Gallstones can also cause inflammation in and obstruction of the bile ducts, leading to a painful condition known as *acute cholecystitis.* Studies have shown that both turmeric and curcumin can help prevent and relieve symptoms of acute cholecystitis due to their proven anti-inflammatory properties.

For many centuries, turmeric has been recommended by practitioners of both Ayurvedic and traditional Chinese medicine (TCM) as a remedy to prevent gallstone formation and relieve their symptoms when they occur. Western science has confirmed turmeric's ability to do so and discovered the reasons why turmeric, along with curcumin, is effective in this regard. First, both turmeric and curcumin stimulate bile production in both the gallbladder and its bile ducts, and also stimulate gallbladder contractions. This helps to maintain proper bile flow. Additionally, as the gallbladder contracts, bile is emptied out from it. This, in turn, helps prevent the buildup of bile and other compounds from combining together to form gallstones.

Turmeric and curcumin also help to prevent the buildup of high levels of cholesterol in bile. Just as importantly, turmeric and curcumin also slow down the time it takes for cholesterol to crystallize. Crystallization of cholesterol is necessary before gallstones can form. Finally, studies have found that limonene, another compound contained in turmeric, is actually capable of dissolving gallstones.

Hemorrhoids

Hemorrhoids are a condition closely related to varicose veins. They are characterized by enlarged, swollen veins that occur within the area of the rectum and anus. They can be both internal (located inside the anus and rectum) or external (located outside the anal cavity). Hemorrhoids are a common gastrointestinal problem, with researchers estimating that as many as 75 percent of all people will develop hemorrhoids at some point in their lives.

In some cases, hemorrhoids are painless and do not present any other symptoms. In other cases, they can not only cause pain, but also bleeding as a result of elimination of stool, as well as itching and burning sensations in and around the areas in which they are present.

The most common treatments for hemorrhoids are a fiber-rich diet along with plenty of water throughout the day, to improve elimination and reduce the risk of straining during bowel movements, and hemorrhoid creams to relieve pain, burning, and itching. Under certain conditions, hemorrhoid pain can become severe and constant enough to warrant surgery. Conventional surgical procedures include the removal of hemorrhoids (hemorrhoidectomy); laser therapy to burn them away; sclerotherapy, or the injection of chemicals into the hemorrhoidal blood supply in order to shrink them; and rubber band ligation or procedure for prolapse and hemorrhoids (PPH), two methods that cut off the blood supply to hemorrhoids so that they shrink. All of these procedures carry the risk of infection, tissue damage, and other complications.

Although people who suffer from hemorrhoids are often told by their doctors to avoid spicy foods, recent research indicates that certain spices, including turmeric, may actually improve hemorrhoid symptoms. Research has found that turmeric's anti-inflammatory properties can help relieve hemorrhoid pain and, in combination with the antibacterial properties turmeric also possesses, can help shrink and heal hemorrhoids when applied topically as an ointment. In Ayurvedic medicine, a common turmeric ointment for hemorrhoids is made from combining dried turmeric powder with ghee (clarified butter) in a ratio of one-to-two; for example, half a teaspoon of turmeric mixed with one teaspoon of ghee. This makes a paste that can be applied topically in and around external hemorrhoid sites at bedtime. (If you choose to try this remedy, be aware that turmeric can stain any cloth it comes in contact with.)

Research has also demonstrated that turmeric can reduce pain and improve the outcomes of pain following surgery to treat hemorrhoids. For example, in one twelve-month study of sixty-seven patients who had received PPH surgery, which involves stapling hemorrhoids to cut off their blood supply, the patients were randomly divided into two groups and matched for the severity of their hemorrhoids, their age, the medications they were on, and other factors. The first group was assigned a bland diet over the twelve-month period, while the other group was assigned a diet that contained turmeric. Over the course of the study, those in the turmeric group required less pain medication and also experienced significantly better overall recoveries.

Another study examined patients who either had a hemorrhoidectomy or an Ayurvedic surgical procedure known as *kshara sutra* ligation, which is similar to rubber band ligation. The difference is that, instead of rubber bands, this procedure uses turmeric-coated suture thread. After both types of surgeries were performed, the hemorrhoidectomy patients were administered antibiotics and pain medication, while the kshara sutra ligation patients were treated with an herbal ointment containing turmeric. The researchers who studied both groups of patients found that 100 percent of the kshara sutra patients were cured of their hemorrhoids, whereas approximately 42 percent of the patients who received an hemorrhoidectomy showed no improvement whatsoever. Moreover, in the kshara sutra group, healing occurred within three to four days, compared to about fourteen days in the hemorrhoidectomy and antibiotic-treated group.

Irritable Bowel Syndrome (IBS)

Irritable bowel syndrome (IBS) is similar to, but not the same as, inflammatory bowel disease (IBD), which includes colitis and Crohn's disease. While both IBS and IBD are characterized by chronic inflammation in the GI tract, along with abdominal pain and bowel changes, the inflammation in IBS is limited to the colon and small intestine. Colitis occurs in the colon and rectum, and Crohn's disease can occur anywhere within the GI tract. In addition, unlike IBD, IBS does not increase the risk for colorectal cancer, and also does not cause abnormal changes to bowel structure.

The primary symptoms of IBS are alternative bouts of constipation and diarrhea caused by pro-inflammatory compounds that affect the enteric nervous system, causing it to signal the brain that something in the GI tract is "wrong." Once the brain receives such signals, it either triggers increased peristalsis in the colon or small intestine, leading to diarrhea, or abnormally slows peristalsis, leading to chronic constipation. Other symptoms of IBS include abdominal pain, bloating, and cramping.

Scientists estimate that as many as 20 percent of all Americans suffer from some degree of IBS. Because the occurrence of its symptoms, especially diarrhea, are so difficult to predict, socializing with others, travel plans, and in many cases, general everyday activities, can be a struggle to manage. In severe cases, people with IBS need to know at all times where the nearest restroom is located when they venture outside of their homes.

Research has shown that turmeric and curcumin can provide relief for people who suffer from IBS. A significant part of the reason that they can do so, of course, has to do with their anti-inflammatory properties. By preventing and reducing inflammation in the GI tract, both compounds can reduce the occurrence and lessen the severity of IBS, as well as reduce associated abdominal pain. In addition, turmeric and curcumin have both been shown to be capable of regulating the body's immune response, thus helping to prevent it from "overreacting" and triggering IBS symptoms. And, because turmeric and curcumin help to regulate overall peristalsis in the GI tract, they can help reduce the incidence of diarrhea and constipation. Finally, overstimulation and angiogenesis of the smallest blood vessels in the intestines can also cause or exacerbate IBS in much the same way that angiogenesis affects inflammatory bowel disease. As you learned in the section on colitis and Crohn's disease, turmeric and curcumin help prevent abnormal angiogenesis in the intestines.

Curcumin supplements can be especially helpful for patients with IBS. An example of curcumin's benefits was demonstrated in the following eight-week study, which involved 200 people with IBS. Their overall IBS symptoms were assessed before, during, and after the study.

The participants were divided into two groups. Each group was given a daily curcumin supplement. The dose for the first group was 72 mg of curcumin, while the second group received double that amount (144 mg). Midway into the study, both groups experienced a significant decrease in the occurrence of their IBS symptoms. The group receiving the lower dose of curcumin exhibited a 53-percent decrease in occurrence, while the group receiving the higher dose exhibited a 60-percent decrease. Both groups also experienced a reduction of their abdominal pain (22 and 25 percent, respectively).

Liver and Pancreas Problems

In order for your body to maintain good health, both your liver and pancreas need to be able to optimally function. Your liver, in particular, is one of the most important organs in your body. It's also one of the most overworked, since it is responsible for performing over 500 essential functions, including:

- breaking down food and aiding your body's assimilation of vital nutrients, manufacturing important hormones such as estrogen and testosterone.

- converting glucose into glycogen, your body's primary energy source.

- fighting infections.

- filtering out toxins and other harmful substances from the nearly 100 gallons of blood that passes through it each day.

- manufacturing bile (an entire quart each day) to break down fat.

- manufacturing healthy cholesterol.

- producing over 13,000 essential chemicals.

- producing urea, which plays an important role helping your body excrete nitrogen.

- regulating blood levels of amino acids, glucose, and fats.

- regulating more than 50,000 vital enzymes, storing essential nutrients, including vitamins A, B_{12}, D, and K.

Your liver is also one of the most important organs for detoxification of both internal waste products and external environmental pollutants. If the liver's ability to detoxify ceased, you would be dead within a matter of hours. However, due to the continued proliferation of environmental toxins, along with common lifestyle factors such as poor diet, alcohol consumption, the regular use of pharmaceutical drugs, and other factors, your liver is constantly under siege. Over time, the impact of these and other factors can result in impaired liver function, setting the stage for poor health.

Your pancreas is an important organ in your body's digestive, endocrine, and immune systems. When healthy, the pancreas produces various enzymes that help digest foods and aid the absorption of fluids and nutrients by the small and large intestines. Some of these enzymes, especially chymotrypsin, also play a role in maintaining your body's immune functions. They are absorbed intact into the bloodstream to be carried to distant body sites, where they digest the fibrin coating on the surface of microbes, cancer cells, and other diseased cells. This allows immune cells to recognize and destroy diseased ones once their protective coating is eliminated.

The pancreas is also the producer of insulin, making this vital organ responsible for balancing blood sugar (glucose) levels in the body. A sufficient supply of glucose to the cells in the body is essential—without this, the cells starve.

According to herbal medicine, both turmeric and curcumin act as natural cholagogues, meaning they stimulate bile production in the liver and encourage excretion of bile. The secretion of bile is vitally important to the whole digestive and assimilative process, particularly with regard to facilitating the digestion of fats. Bile produced in the liver, as well as in the gallbladder, also acts as a natural laxative, helping the liver perform its many detoxification functions.

Both turmeric and curcumin also help the liver convert the cholesterol it produces into bile acids, both by stimulating an enzyme known as hepatic cholesterol-7-alpha-hydroxylase, which plays a primary role in bile acid synthesis, and through increased bile acid secretion itself. This, in turn, helps keep cholesterol levels in check. Research has also demonstrated that turmeric and curcumin help protect the liver from various toxins and infections. Because of this, they can also protect against liver conditions such as hepatitis, jaundice, and cirrhosis. They also offer further protection against such conditions because of their ability to prevent the liver's hepatic ducts from becoming swollen and bloated, and for their ability to shrink these ducts when they are engorged. In this regard, turmeric and curcumin offer similar liver-protective benefits as milk thistle and artichoke leaves, two more common herbal remedies that are often prescribed here in the United States.

Because of the way they support the ability of the pancreas to manufacture and secrete its digestive and immune-bolstering enzymes, turmeric and curcumin are both effective natural remedies in helping to maintain healthy pancreatic function. Researchers have found that turmeric and curcumin both increase production of amylase, lipase, trypsin, and chymotrypsin. As a result, they are also helpful natural aids in improving and maintaining overall digestive, endocrine, and immune function.

Ulcers

Ulcers and gastritis are common GI conditions. They are typically caused by a number of different factors, often in combination with each other, all of which create both inflammation and an imbalance in the pH level in the stomach. Symptoms of ulcers and gastritis include stomach pain, burning sensations in the stomach, and pain after eating or lying down. In some cases, ulcers can cause the stomach lining to weaken or bleed. If not treated in time, this can lead to death.

One of the most common causes is the presence of the bacteria *Helicobacter pylori* (H. pylori) in the stomach. Despite the stomach's normally highly acidic environment, H. pylori bacteria are able to survive because they form a protective coating called a biofilm. Eliminating H. pylori can dramatically reduce the high risk of a recurrence of ulcers and gastritis.

Research shows that turmeric and curcumin are both effective natural remedies for preventing ulcers and gastritis, and can also be helpful for treating and healing both conditions. Additional research has shown that curcumin supplements taken with anti-ulcer drugs can improve the effectiveness of such drugs.

In large part, the ulcer- and gastritis-healing benefits turmeric and curcumin provide have to do with their anti-inflammatory, antioxidant, and antimicrobial properties, all of which can improve stomach health and inhibit the conditions in the stomach that can cause ulcers and gastritis. In addition, research has also found that turmeric and curcumin provide benefits that anti-ulcer drugs do not provide. These important benefits include regulating the enzymes associated with ulcers, reverse cell damage in the stomach, and accelerating the healing of ulcerous wounds. Curcumin and other compounds found in turmeric also inhibit the secretion of gastric acids, block histamine receptors that trigger inflammation, increase mucus, and aid in the restoration of normal biochemical activities in the stomach, all without the risk of the side effects that are commonly caused by anti-ulcer drugs.

Clinical studies have also found that turmeric and curcumin block the growth and spread of H. pylori and prevent the bacteria from activating NF-κB. This, in turn, prevents NF-κB from triggering the genes that produce inflammation-causing cytokines within the stomach. Researchers have also found that turmeric and curcumin can significantly delay the formation of the biofilm that otherwise protects H. pylori, further inhibiting the bacteria's ability to grow and spread in the stomach.

Research with animals has also shown that turmeric and curcumin are able to more effectively regulate enzyme activity and increase the rate of healing of stomach ulcers compared to the anti-ulcer drug omeprazole (Prilosec). Other research has found that turmeric contains various other compounds that possess anti-ulcer properties. One of these, caffeic acid, has been shown to suppress the activity of MMP-9 (*Matrix Metalloproteinase-9*), an enzyme that not only promotes the growth of ulcers but also inhibits them from healing. Caffeic acid has also been shown to reduce the pain that stomach ulcers can cause.

The benefits that turmeric and curcumin provide for preventing and healing ulcers can be seen in the following studies. The first study involved fifty-five men and women, all of whom had peptic ulcers. Thirty-five of the study participants also tested positive for H. pylori at the beginning of the study. All of the participants we given an oral turmeric extract supplement (500 mg) four times a day, an hour before their meals. Within four weeks, the ulcers of thirty-five of the fifty-five patients were completely healed, and by the end of the second month this number increased to forty-seven. In addition, by the end of the study, twenty of the thirty-five patients who had tested positive for H. pylori were free of the bacteria.

In a second study, forty-five men and women were tested. Twenty-five of them were confirmed to have peptic ulcers after receiving endoscopies, while the remaining twenty participants had gastritis and were in the early stages of developing ulcers. All of the participants were given oral turmeric supplements five times a day (600 mg per dose). The supplements were taken thirty to sixty minutes before meals, then at 4 PM, and then just before bedtime. By the end of four weeks, 48 percent of the participants achieved complete healing of their ulcers, and by the end of twelve weeks, this increased to 76 percent of the participants.

Based on the above information and study findings, you now have a clearer understanding of how and why turmeric and curcumin can not only improve and maintain your digestion, but can also protect you from the most common gastrointestinal conditions, some of which can be quite serious.

OTHER STEPS YOU CAN TAKE
TO MAINTAIN A HEALTHY GI TRACT

In addition to using turmeric to spice up your meals and taking a daily curcumin supplement, here are other steps you can take that will help improve your digestion and the overall functioning of your GI tract:

1. Emphasize a whole foods diet that includes plenty of fresh, organic fruits and vegetables and fiber-rich foods. Also reduce your intake of high-carbohydrate foods, and avoid all processed foods, food additives and preservatives, unhealthy fats, and sugar. For some people, eliminating coffee and other caffeine products may also be necessary. Similarly, while a glass of wine or beer can often aid digestion for some people, others may need to avoid such beverages. All other forms of alcohol should also be eliminated.

2. Drink plenty of pure, filtered water throughout the day, but avoid drinking water with your meals. Ideally, have water twenty minutes before or at least an hour after you eat, because water taken with meals can interfere with digestion.

3. If you suffer from chronic indigestion or other GI problems, consider being checked for food allergies and sensitivities, parasites, and bacterial, fungal, or viral infections, all of which can contribute to leaky gut syndrome and provoke autoimmune reactions. To do so, seek out physicians trained in environmental medicine.

4. Consider the use of probiotics and the use of soil-based organisms (SBOs) to restore a healthy balance to the intestinal flora. Also consider adding fermented foods such as sauerkraut, miso soup, and kimchi to your diet, as such foods can significantly boost the level of healthy bacteria in your gut.

5. Learn how to manage stress, and become aware of various triggers in your life that can cause you to feel stressed. Also seek help if you need to heal anger and other debilitating or suppressed emotions, and try not to eat when you are emotionally agitated. All these factors can cause or exacerbate GI problems.

6. To further aid your digestion, consider taking digestive enzymes with your meals. Supplementing with hydrochloric acid (HCl) tablets can also be helpful, especially before eating protein-rich foods. HCl is produced in the stomach and is essential for the proper digestion of protein. As we age, however, our bodies typically produced less HCl.

7. Try to engage in moderate exercise on a regular basis. Doing so can aid digestion and helps promote healthy and regular bowel movements. If possible, try to take a twenty to thirty minute walk each day after your largest meal.

8. Avoid eating after 8 PM, and ideally even earlier, as late meals can interfere with your ability to achieve a good night's sleep and are more likely to be poorly digested.

CONCLUSION

Having read this chapter, you now have a better idea as to why good digestion and a properly functioning GI tract are so important to both your physical and mental/emotional health. You've also learned how and why the regular use of turmeric as a spice added to your meals, along with taking a daily curcumin supplement, can go a long way towards improving your digestion and protecting your body's GI tract. These two simple steps are easy to implement, and I encourage you to do so.

In the next chapter, you will discover how and why turmeric and curcumin can help prevent arthritis and other types of joint pain.

7

Turmeric & Arthritis

*A*rthritis is a blanket term for more than 100 disease conditions of the musculoskeletal system that affect the joints, tendons, ligaments, and cartilage. The term itself is derived from the Greek words *artho,* which means "joint," and *itis,* which refers to inflammation. Arthritis is one of the oldest and most common forms of all diseases, and affects approximately 15 percent of all Americans, making it the leading cause of disability in the United States.

Typically, arthritis is more likely to occur as we age, but it can strike anyone, including children. In the United States, it is estimated that approximately 40 percent of all people over sixty-five have arthritis to some degree. While arthritis can affect any joint in the body, it most commonly affects the fingers, knees, and hips.

The most prevalent type of arthritis is osteoarthritis, an inflammatory joint disease that, over time, causes a breakdown in the cartilage covering the bone inside the joint. The primary symptoms of osteoarthritis are pain, stiffness, and joint swelling. Rheumatoid arthritis is less common than osteoarthritis and afflicts primarily women. It is an autoimmune disease, meaning that it is caused by the immune system attacking its own tissues. It affects the membrane lining the body's joints, known as *synovial tissue.* The primary function of this tissue is to secrete lubricant so that bones can move against each other without pain. The joints of people suffering from rheumatoid arthritis are tender and swollen, and can sometimes become deformed. Additional symptoms include depression, lethargy, and night sweats. Another common type of arthritis is gout, caused by excess uric acid buildup in the body that usually first manifests in the toes, especially the big toe.

There are no definitive diagnostic tests for arthritis, and conventional treatment of the disease is primarily aimed at treating symptoms. Conventional care includes reduction of joint stress, physical therapy such as exercise, hot and cold packs, diathermy (the use of electrically induced heat or high-frequency electromagnetic currents as a form of physical or occupational therapy), drugs (especially prescription and over-the-counter pain relief drugs, such as aspirin and other analgesics, and nonsteroidal anti-inflammatory drugs, or NSAIDs, such as ibuprofen), and, as a late-stage intervention, surgery (including reconstruction or replacement of affected joints).

Among the risk factors for arthritis are heredity, being overweight (total body weight and body mass index are significant predictors of osteoarthritis in the knee, for instance), lack of or excessive exercise (particularly exercises such as long-distance running and basketball, which result in violent joint-pounding), joint injury, skeletal postural defects, and joint instability. While arthritic symptoms may be limited to a particular joint, it is important to realize that, like all other chronic conditions, it is a *systemic disease,* meaning that it affects the whole body and is usually associated with other systemic disorders. These can include digestive imbalances, nutritional deficiencies, endocrine disorders, and low-grade infection. In addition, arthritis sufferers commonly have an excess of acid in the body. These acidic toxins can be deposited in the joints, leading to inflammation and pain.

Overall, conventional medical treatments for arthritis have a very poor record when it comes to reversing it. At best, such treatments only offer temporary relief of arthritis symptoms, while failing to truly address the underlying causes that are associated with arthritic conditions. As a result, arthritis patients prescribed medications to manage their symptoms typically are required to continue taking such drugs long-term. But long-term use of the same drugs usually results in diminished pain relief. More importantly, continued use of such drugs is known to cause severe health problems, such as immune system disorders, serious gastrointestinal complications, and cardiovascular conditions, including death by heart attack and stroke.

In fact, as a result of these health risks, the Food and Drug Administration (FDA) has been forced to withdraw a number of these arthritis drugs after it first approved them. The most infamous example of this is the arthritis drug Vioxx, which was taken off the market after the FDA estimated that it contributed to 27,785 heart attacks and sudden cardiac deaths between 1999 and 2003, and tripled the risk of death from both of these diseases by 300 percent. Other researchers estimate the number of deaths caused by Vioxx was much higher, possibly 60,000 or more. Vioxx was pulled from the marketplace in 2004.

Fortunately, scientists have discovered that both turmeric and curcumin provide the same advantages for arthritis sufferers that arthritis medications do, and offer more benefits than single-action drugs. Moreover, they are safe to use for extended periods of time, if necessary, without the fear of harmful side effects.

HOW AND WHY TURMERIC CAN PREVENT AND HELP REVERSE ARTHRITIS

By now, having read this far in the book, you likely realize that it is the ability of turmeric and curcumin to significantly reduce levels of inflammation in the body, that is a major reason why these substances can act as such potent natural aids in preventing and reversing arthritis. Simply put, inflammation causes pain, including arthritis pain, and eliminating or reducing inflammation gets rid of pain.

As you learned in Chapter 6, clinical studies have proven that turmeric and curcumin inhibit the pro-inflammatory activity of a protein complex known as NF-κB, a primary activator of inflammation in the immune system that is also known to trigger genes to produce various other inflammatory substances, including COX-2 enzymes. The reduction of COX-2 enzymes can significantly reduce the pain caused by arthritis. It is for this reason that NSAID drugs are so commonly prescribed for arthritis patients. Such drugs acts as COX-2 inhibitors. However, as mentioned, these drugs also carry a very high risk for serious, even life-threatening side effects, whereas the use of turmeric and curcumin has been proven by researchers to be extremely safe.

As you also learned in the last chapter, caffeic acid, one of the other compounds found in turmeric, has been shown to suppress the activity of MMP-9 (*Matrix Metalloproteinase-9*), which can also cause inflammation and pain. Researchers have found that turmeric, and especially curcumin taken as an oral supplement, can reduce COX-2 enzymes, MMP-9, and various others of the body's pro-inflammatory triggers, such as cytokines, by as much as 99 percent. Such a significant reduction translates to nearly complete relief of chronic pain.

There are other important reasons besides their anti-inflammatory properties that also explain why both turmeric and curcumin should be considered for preventing and relieving arthritis symptoms. Another significant factor is their proven antioxidant effects. Clinical studies have well-established that turmeric and curcumin can both reduce the harmful effects of oxidative stress on their own, while also increasing the activities of other antioxidants in the body, such as superoxide dismutase (SOD) and glutathione.

Turmeric's and curcumin's mechanisms of action with regard to their antioxidant properties all can be helpful for preventing and taming arthritis pain. Not only have they been shown to scavenge and neutralize different types of free radicals, such as reactive oxygen species (ROS) and reactive nitrogen species (RNS), they also enhance the ability of SOD enzymes and glutathione to defuse free radicals. Furthermore, turmeric and curcumin act as lipophilic compounds, meaning they are capable of dissolving lipids (fats), operating as efficient scavengers of lipid-based free radicals, such as peroxyls. In this capacity, they act similarly to vitamin C and vitamin E as chain-breaking antioxidants.

Finally, studies have shown that turmeric and curcumin offer another very important benefit for arthritis sufferers. Both of them not only help prevent the breakdown of cartilage that is associated with osteoarthritis, as well as other musculoskeletal disorders, but can also help build new cartilage cells. Thus they are capable of not only stopping cartilage deterioration but also reversing it.

The following studies illustrate just how effective turmeric and curcumin can be for relieving both osteo- and rheumatoid arthritis pain, as well as other symptoms.

Comparing Turmeric to Ibuprofen

The first study was a clinical trial of 367 patients suffering from osteoarthritis in their knees. On a scale of one to ten, with ten being the highest level of pain, all of the participants' pain scores were greater than five. The purpose of this study was to compare turmeric extracts to ibuprofen in terms of their effectiveness for alleviating the participants' knee pain. The participants were randomly divided into two groups. 185 patients received the turmeric extract once a day for four week, at a dose of 1,500 mg/day. The remaining 182 patients were administered ibuprofen once a day for the same time period, as a dose of 1,200 mg/day.

At the beginning of the study, its authors reported that the "baseline characteristics were no different between groups," meaning that both groups were comprised of people with the same degrees of pain and other overall symptoms. Before, during, and at the study's conclusion, both groups of participants were evaluated using Western Ontario and McMaster Universities Osteoarthritis Index (WOMAC) total, WOMAC pain, WOMAC stiffness, and WOMAC function scores. (WOMAC scores are a common means of assessing the degree of symptoms associated with osteoarthritis.) The incidence of adverse events (AE) within each group were also closely monitored.

According to the study's authors, by the second week of the study and at its conclusion after week four, the WOMAC scores in both groups showed "significant improvement when compared with the baseline" of both groups at the beginning of the study. More importantly, the study found that the turmeric extract was equally effective as ibuprofen for treating knee pain caused by osteoarthritis. The authors of the study also wrote, "The number of patients who developed AEs was no different between groups. However, the number of events of abdominal pain/discomfort was significantly higher in the ibuprofen group." This, too, is significant, because it reveals that not only are turmeric extracts as good as ibuprofen for treating osteoarthritis knee pain, but are also much safer, and thus far more suitable for long-term use than ibuprofen is.

Comparing Curcumin to Acetaminophen and Nimesulide

Another study also demonstrated curcumin's pain relief properties, although not specifically for pain caused by arthritis. The participants in this study all suffered from acute pain. They were divided into different groups. One group received Meriva, a curcumin formula made with lecithin at different dose levels (2,000 mg of Meriva containing 400 mg of curcumin and 1,500 mg of Meriva containing 300 mg of curcumin, respectively), while another group was administered acetaminophen (Tylenol) at a standard dose of 500 mg. A third group was given the NSAID drug nimesulide, which acts as a COX-2 inhibitor at a dose of 100 mg.

The participants in the study who received Meriva containing the higher dose of curcumin experienced greater pain relief compared to those who received acetaminophen. According to researchers, the pain relief offered by Meriva at this dose was comparable to that offered by acetaminophen taken at a dose of 1,000 mg. Meriva was not as effective as nimesulide, however. Additionally, those who received Meriva with the lower dose of curcumin experienced only fleeting, reduced pain relief compared to the acetaminophen and nimesulfide groups.

Moreover, participants taking Meriva with the higher dose of curcumin achieved significant pain relief within two hours after it was administered, which was similar in duration to acetaminophen. Nimesulfide achieved the fastest acting effects, with pain relief being achieved within one hour after it was administered. However, the patients who were given nimesulfide also experienced significant gastrointestinal problems as a side effect of the drug, whereas neither the Meriva nor the acetaminophen groups experienced such symptoms.

As a result of this study, the authors wrote, "Taken together, our results show that the preclinical analgesic [pain relief] properties of curcumin have clinical relevance, at least at a dose of 2 g[rams] as the Meriva formulation. . . . In patients on treatment with Meriva, this would also translate into better control of acute pain."

Treating Knee Pain with Curcuminoids

Other studies have also confirmed the effectiveness of turmeric and curcumin for treating knee pain caused by osteoarthritis. In one of them, which was also a randomized, double-blind, placebo-controlled trial, forty test subjects with knee pain ranging from mild to moderate were randomly divided into two groups. The first group received 500 mg/day of curcuminoid in three divided doses, along with 5 mg piperine added to each 500-mg dose to improve its absorption. Piperine is the active ingredient in black pepper. In India and other countries where turmeric is commonly used, black pepper is also used at the same time for this reason, as well as for the flavoring both spices provide to foods. The other group received a matched placebo each day. The study lasted for six weeks.

As in the previous study, the participants were assessed using WOMAC scores, as well as two other measurements, one known as the visual analog scale (VAS), the other called the Lequesne's pain functional index (LPFI). At the end of the study, the participants who received curcuminoid exhibited "significantly greater reductions" in their VAS, WOMAC, and LPFI scores compared to the placebo group, with especially notable improvement in their pain and physical function scores, with the exception of stiffness, which remained similar to that of the placebo group. In addition, blood testing revealed that the curcuminoid group also achieved a decrease in their bodies' overall levels of oxidative stress, whereas there were no such improvements in the placebo group.

Interestingly, the researchers of this study also found that the improvements achieved by the curcuminoid group in their pain and physical function scores were not due to changes in circulating cytokines. The authors suggested that this lack of change, coupled with the participants' improved pain scores, have been because in cases of osteoarthritis, it is more likely that changes in the inflammatory markers within synovial fluid, and not the rest of the body, are elevated. (Synovial fluid acts as a lubricant to prevent friction in the bones of the knees and other joints.) This is different than cases of rheumatoid arthritis, in which there is a systemic (body-wide) increase in inflammatory markers, including cytokines.

Based on their findings and observations, the authors wrote that the beneficial effects of curcuminoids for osteoarthritis pain may be because these effects are localized, meaning they directly target areas of pain in the body. However, they also added that the time period of the study may not have been long enough to determine this for certain. Either way, their findings furthered confirmed that curcumin extracts, and therefore curcumin itself, are effective in relieving pain and improving physical functioning in patients suffering from osteoarthritis knee pain, while also reducing overall oxidative stress in the body.

Treating Osteoarthritis with Turmeric Extracts

In a much longer randomized, double blind study that lasted for eight months, fifty patients diagnosed with osteoarthritis were divided into two groups. The first group received standard conventional medical care as by their physician, while the second group also received standard care along with a twice-daily dose (500 mg each time) of a natural supplement comprised of turmeric extracts, phosphatidyl-choline, and microcrystalline cellulose. Both groups were tested before, during, and after the study, using WOMAC scores and measurements of their physical function and stiffness levels.

By the end of the study, the group who received the natural supplement along with standard conventional care showed significant decreases in all of the above scores and measurement levels compared to the group receiving only conventional medical care. In addition, and just as importantly, the participants receiving the supplement containing turmeric extracts also showed significant decreases in all of their markers for chronic inflammation. There was no decrease at all in these markers within the other group of participants.

The authors of a meta-analysis that examined a number of other studies showing the benefits that both turmeric and curcumin have in relieving osteoarthritis pain and other related symptoms wrote, "Regardless of the mechanism by which curcumin elicits its effects, it does appear to be beneficial to several aspects of OA [osteoarthritis], as suggested by a recent systematic review and meta-analysis that concluded: 'This systematic review and meta-analysis provided scientific evidence that eight to twelve weeks of standardized turmeric extracts (typically 1000 mg/day of curcumin) treatment can reduce arthritis symptoms (mainly pain and inflammation-related symptoms) and result in similar improvements in the symptoms as ibuprofen and diclofenac sodium [another NSAID to which turmeric extracts and curcumin were compared]. Therefore, turmeric extracts and curcumin can be recommended for alleviating the symptoms of arthritis, especially osteoarthritis.'"

Treating Rheumatoid Arthritis with Turmeric

Turmeric and curcumin have also been shown to offer benefits for people suffering with rheumatoid arthritis (RA). An animal study, for example, has found that turmeric offers superior relief of RA symptoms compared to indomethacin, an NSAID medication commonly prescribed to manage rheumatoid arthritis, as well as ginger, another herb that is often used to treat RA.

In this study, rats were induced by scientists to develop RA, after which they were given either turmeric, ginger, or indomethacin. The authors of the study wrote:

> Both plants [turmeric and ginger] (at dose 200 mg/kg body weight) significantly suppressed (but with different degrees) the incidence and severity of arthritis by increasing/decreasing the production of anti-inflammatory/pro-inflammatory cytokines, respectively, and activating the anti-oxidant defense system. The anti-arthritic activity of turmeric exceeded that of ginger and indomethacin (a non-steroidal anti-inflammatory drug), especially when the treatment started from the day of arthritis induction. . . . The present study proves the anti-inflammatory/anti-oxidant activity of turmeric over ginger and indomethacin, which may have beneficial effects against rheumatoid arthritis onset/progression."

In a different study, researchers investigated the potential that curcumin and cyclocurcumin, a curcumin derivative, have for treating rheumatoid arthritis. The authors of the study wrote, "We focused on prominent p38 mitogen-activated protein (MAP) kinase p38α which is a prime regulator of tumor necrosis factor-α (TNF-α), a key mediator of rheumatoid arthritis," adding that, "[t]he overexpression of tumor necrosis factor-α (TNF-α) is a prime inflammatory cascade involved in RA. This cascade leads to the overexpression of cytokines such as interleukin-1 (IL-1), IL-6 and IL-10, which drives persistent inflammation and joint destruction."

In the study, the researchers examined how curcumin and its derivative bind with active p38α sites in the body. "Targeting of p38α has demonstrated efficacy in animal models of RA and various p38α inhibitors are currently in phase II and I clinical trials for RA," they explained. "Thus using p38α as a therapeutic target for the development of a novel compound is a viable option." Their findings "confirmed strong inhibition of p38α by curcumin," and, just as importantly, showed that curcumin and cyclocurcumin inhibited the release of TNF-α from human macrophages, a class of immune cells. This is significant because, as the authors wrote, "TNF-α is a key factor in a variety of inflammatory diseases," including rheumatoid arthritis.

As the authors of this study also pointed out, "Curcumin has long been reported to have an antirheumatoid effect." They concluded their study by writing that their findings demonstrated that "the potential binding mode of cyclocurcumin with p38α with stability was revealed as a top compound for the treatment of RA [rheumatoid arthritis]. Finally, inhibition of the release of TNF-α from LPS-stimulated macrophages by cyclocurcumin treatment confirms its role as a potent p38α inhibitor."

Another study demonstrated that curcumin can counteract the effects of inflammatory agents known as synoviocytes in both joint and the synovial fluid that surrounds them. Inflammation in the synovial fluid and joints is primary cause of rheumatoid arthritis, and synoviocytes are known to trigger that inflammation. And, as it does with p38α mentioned in the study above, the release of tumor necrosis factor-α (TNF-α) plays a major role that causes synoviocytes to become inflammatory.

For this study, researchers stimulated synoviocytes with TNF-α The researchers found that these synoviocytes treated with curcumin mitigated the harmful effects caused by TNF-α, and reversed them to "a considerable extent." Moreover, curcumin was also found to improve the metabolism of both amino acids (glycine, citrulline, arachidonic acid) and saturated fatty acids within the synoviocytes. It is this restorative effect, the researchers speculated, that may better explain how and why curcumin is known to be effective in preventing and relieving joint inflammation.

A pilot study published in 2012 further demonstrated curcumin's effectiveness for managing the symptoms of rheumatoid arthritis, as well as its safety as a treatment for RA. In the study, which consisted of forty-five patients with RA, the subjects were randomly divided into three groups. The first group received curcumin at a dose of 500 mg, the second group received a standard dose (50 mg), while the third group received both curcumin and diclofenac sodium, an NSAID. The patients in all three groups were assessed using what is known as a Disease Activity Score 28 (DAS), along with the American College of Rheumatology's (ACR) criteria for reduction in tenderness and swelling of joint scores.

"Patients in all three treatment groups showed statistically significant changes in their DAS scores," the authors of this study wrote. "Interestingly, the curcumin group showed the highest percentage of improvement in overall DAS and ACR scores (ACR 20, 50 and 70) and these scores were significantly better than the patients in the diclofenac sodium group. More importantly, curcumin treatment was found to be safe and did not relate with any adverse events. Our study provides the first evidence for the safety and superiority of curcumin treatment in patients with active RA, and highlights the need for future large-scale trials to validate these findings in patients with RA and other arthritic conditions."

The findings of the above and other studies gained further support from a 2017 study published in the scientific *Journal of Medicinal Food*. The published abstract of this study speaks for itself:

Rheumatoid arthritis (RA) is an autoimmune, chronic systemic inflammatory disorder. The long-term use of currently available drugs for the treatment of RA has many potential side effects. Natural phytonutrients may serve as alternative strategies for the safe and effective treatment of RA, and curcuminoids have been used in Ayurvedic medicine for the treatment of inflammatory conditions for centuries.

In this study, a novel, highly bioavailable form of curcumin in a completely natural turmeric matrix was evaluated for its ability to improve the clinical symptoms of RA. A randomized, double-blind, placebo-controlled, three-arm, parallel-group study was conducted to evaluate the comparative efficacy of two different doses of curcumin with that of a placebo in active RA patients. Twelve patients in each group received placebo, 250 mg, or 500 mg of the curcumin product twice daily for ninety days.

The responses of the patients were assessed using the American College of Rheumatology (ACR) response, visual analog scale (VAS), C-reactive protein (CRP), Disease Activity Score 28 (DAS28), erythrocyte sedimentation rate (ESR), and rheumatoid factor (RF) values. RA patients who received the curcumin product at both low and high doses reported statistically significant changes in their clinical symptoms at the end of the study. These observations were confirmed by significant changes in ESR, CPR, and RF values in patients receiving the study product compared to baseline and placebo.

The results indicate that this novel curcumin in a turmeric matrix acts as an analgesic and anti-inflammatory agent for the management of RA at a dose as low as 250 mg twice daily, as evidenced by significant improvement in the ESR, CRP, VAS, RF, DAS28, and ACR responses compared to placebo. Both doses of the study product were well tolerated and without side effects.

The above studies are but a sampling of all the research that has been conducted that confirms the ability of curcumin and other compounds found in turmeric to provide significant relief of arthritic pain and other arthritis symptoms, and in helping prevent arthritis (both osteo- and rheumatoid) from developing in the first place. This is also true for other types of joint pain, such as ankle sprains, as well as such conditions such as back, neck, or shoulder pain. If you suffer from any of these conditions, you may be pleasantly surprised by how much turmeric, and especially curcumin, can help you.

STEPS YOU CAN TAKE
TO PREVENT AND REVERSE ARTHRITIS

Like most other chronic, degenerative diseases, arthritis in its many forms is caused by a variety of underlying and interrelated issues, all of which can combine together to trigger inflammation and its associated co-factors that cause and exacerbate it.

The first and perhaps most important step you can take is to adopt an anti-inflammatory diet that not only reduces levels of inflammation in your body, but also does not force it to draw upon its stores of alkalizing minerals (calcium, magnesium, and potassium) in order to manage the damaging effects of too much acidity. In cultures around the world, people consume meals that are rich in alkalizing foods and beverages. Their diets contain low or moderate amounts of foods that create acidic residues in the body once they are digested and metabolized. Such meals contain a plentiful supply of fresh, raw or lightly steamed vegetables, fresh fruits, and grains, along with small portions of fish, poultry, or meat. The key is to try to consume between 60 to 80 percent of foods for each meal that produce an alkalizing effect in the body.

A full discussion of such foods and meal plans is well beyond the scope of this book. If you are interested in learning more about the most alkalizing and acidifying foods and beverages, I recommend *The Acid-Alkaline Food Guide,* which I co-wrote with Dr. Susan E. Brown, one of the world's foremost experts on the subject.

Also be sure to avoid white flour, sugar, all unhealthy fats (margarine and most vegetable oils, except extra virgin olive oil), and soft drinks, all of which are known triggers for arthritis and many other degenerative diseases. Healthy fats, however, especially omega-3 essential fatty acids found in fish, flaxseed and flaxseed oil, and the medium-chain fatty acids contained in organic, extra virgin coconut, should be included in your diet because they all provide potent, natural anti-inflammatory benefits.

In addition to a healthy diet, other important steps you can take include:

1. Drinking plenty of pure, filtered water each and every day, ideally between meals so as not to dilute your body's ability to properly digest the foods you eat. The late Dr. Fereydoon Batmanghelidj, who during his lifetime was considered the world's foremost expert on the many ways in which water could prevent and reverse a wide range of disease conditions, helped many people completely cure themselves from both osteo- and rheumatoid arthritis simply by increasing their daily water intake. Research conducted by Dr. Batman, as he liked to be called, conclusively proved that

chronic, low-grade dehydration in the body is a primary trigger of chronic inflammation.

2. Certain nutritional supplements in addition to turmeric and curcumin extracts can also be helpful. These include vitamins A, B_1, B_3 (niacin), B_6, C, D, E, and K, omega-3 oils, and the minerals magnesium, sulfur, and especially boron, all of which are lacking in our crop soil, and therefore in the foods grown in it.

3. Losing weight if you need to do so is also important, since excess weight causes increased stress on the joints affected by arthritis, especially the knees and feet.

4. Daily gentle stretching exercises can also be helpful for improving joint mobility and keeping limber.

5. Massage, chiropractic, and other forms of bodywork can also help support the overall health of your body's musculoskeletal system and provide relief to arthritic joints.

CONCLUSION

By reading this chapter, you've gained a better understanding of what causes the various forms of arthritis and learned why conventional drugs for treating it are so often ineffective and even dangerous. You've also learned how and why turmeric and curcumin have proven to be as effective as, and even superior to, such drug treatments, and, because of how valuable both compounds are, can also go a long way toward preventing arthritis. So, if you suffer from arthritis, or have no wish to ever develop it, you now have more important reasons why you should consider regularly adding turmeric as a spice to your meals and taking a high quality curcumin supplement.

In the next chapter, you will discover the benefits turmeric and curcumin offer for helping to prevent and better manage type 2 diabetes.

8

Turmeric & Diabetes

In this chapter, we are going to explore the many important ways in which turmeric and curcumin can help prevent one of the most common health problems affecting many Americans today: diabetes.

There are two main types of diabetes: insulin-dependent juvenile, or Type I diabetes, and non-insulin dependent, more commonly known as Type II diabetes. Both Type I and Type II diabetes are characterized by chronic high blood sugar levels, as well as other disturbances in carbohydrate, fat, and protein metabolism. Type II diabetes is by far the most prevalent form of diabetes, accounting for between 90 and 95 percent of all cases in the United States, and is the form that this chapter is focused on.

WHAT IS TYPE II DIABETES?

Type II diabetes is a chronic, degenerative disease caused by insulin resistance, a condition in which the cells of the body resist insulin's attempts at regulating blood sugar levels. Insulin is a hormone produced by the pancreas to metabolize glucose, a form of sugar that is one of the primary sources of cells' energy supply. When insulin resistance occurs, the body is unable to transport enough glucose, its primary fuel source, from the bloodstream into the cells, especially after meals, when blood sugar levels rise as a natural consequence of digestion.

Normally, blood sugar levels are kept in check by the body's self-regulating mechanisms, known as homeostasis. A rise in blood glucose after eating is supposed to stimulate production of the hormone insulin, and the insulin released into the bloodstream is supposed to keep blood sugar levels within a safe and usable range. In cases of insulin resistance, glucose levels remain high. When this situation becomes chronic, the stage is set for diabetes to occur.

In the past, type II diabetes was often referred to as "late adult onset diabetes" because it typically did not strike adults until they reached their 50s or beyond. However, today type II diabetes is so prevalent that it is occurring even among children and teenagers at an alarming rate. This near-epidemic increase in the incidence of type II diabetes is due to a variety of factors, but the three most common causes being poor diet, obesity, and a sedentary lifestyle. Type II diabetes accounts for nearly 10 percent of all deaths in the United States of people twenty-five and older. It is also the main cause of new cases of blindness among adults between the ages of twenty to seventy-four years old, and it is the leading cause of end-stage kidney disease. In addition, type II diabetes is the primary reason for limb amputations.

Making matters worse, it is estimated that a third of all people who have diabetes are unaware that they do so, while millions of other Americans, including children and teens, are already in a pre-diabetic state that they also are not aware of. Left unchecked, pre-diabetes will inevitably become type II diabetes. Having type II diabetes also significantly increases the risk for heart attack, stroke, and other types of heart disease. People with diabetes, for

---

Testing for Type II Diabetes

Because both type II diabetes and pre-diabetes can so often develop without a person being aware that they are doing so, regular (yearly) testing for these conditions is an important step you can take to safeguard your health.

Pre- and type II diabetes are generally tested for by measuring the amount of glucose in the bloodstream. There are different types of tests that can be used for this purpose. One is a direct measurement of blood glucose levels after an overnight fast, and the second is the measurement of the body's ability to handle excess sugar after drinking liquid glucose.

The most common indicator of diabetes is a recurring elevated blood sugar level after an overnight fast. A fasting blood sugar value above 126 mg/dl on at least two separate occasions is said to be indicative of diabetes (whereas normal values are between 65 and 99 mg/dl, with lower levels within this range being optimal), while recurring blood sugar levels between 100 and 125 are indicative of a pre-diabetic state.

However, a more accurate means of testing for type II diabetes is with a glucose tolerance test that checks both glucose and insulin levels. This test measures how well your body's cells are able to absorb glucose after sugar or other glucose-rich foods are consumed.

example, have a 300- to 400-percent greater risk of dying from heart attacks than people without diabetes who have the same number of other major risk factors. Type II diabetes also increases the risk of cancer as well as other serious health problems. This is why being tested for diabetes is so important.

Classic symptoms of Type II diabetes are excessive thirst, excessive urination, excessive hunger, unhealthy weight gain, and persistent fatigue. Other warning signs include carbohydrate cravings, bouts of dizziness, irritability, progressive weight gain (especially around the waist), an increase in blood triglycerides and cholesterol levels, a progressive increase in blood pressure, fainting episodes, and frequent fungal infections. If you suffer from any of these symptoms, by all means, see your doctor.

HOW TURMERIC AND CURCUMIN CAN HELP PEOPLE WITH TYPE II DIABETES

Both type II diabetes and pre-diabetes are diseases in which both chronic inflammation and oxidative stress (free radical damage) play primary roles. Throughout this book, you've learned how and why turmeric and curcumin

---

As with a standard blood sugar test, before receiving a glucose tolerance test, you will be asked to fast for at least eight hours. At the start of the test, your blood will be drawn to determine your fasting blood glucose level. You will then be asked to drink an eight-ounce glucose syrup containing 75 grams of sugar. You will then wait for two hours, at which time your blood will again be drawn. Blood sugar readings from the second blood draw of between 140 to 199 mg/dL are an indicator of pre-diabetes, while a reading of 200 mg/dL is a confirmation of diabetes.

A third testing method that can also be used to screen for diabetes and pre-diabetes is called the hemoglobin A1c (HbA1c) test. It can help your doctor to determine whether or not damage is being caused to the proteins in your blood as a result of free radicals caused by glucose binding to oxygen-carrying hemoglobin in red blood cells. The results for this test are expressed as a percentage, with normal levels ranging from 4.5 to 4.9 percent. Research indicates that a measurement of HbA1c between 5.7 and 6.9 percent is an indication of pre-diabetes, with readings of 7.0 percent or greater being a sign of diabetes.

This test can also accurately predict your risk of developing a variety of other health problems, including heart attacks. Research has shown that every 1-percent increase in HbA1c increases the risk of heart attack by an average of 20 percent.

can be so effective in both preventing and helping to reverse these disease-triggering mechanisms in the body. Therefore, it's not surprising that research has shown that turmeric and curcumin offer both preventive and therapeutic benefits with regard to type II diabetes and pre-diabetes.

Preventing and Minimizing the Effects of Diabetes

In addition to their ability to counteract inflammation and oxidative stress, studies have also shown that the anti-diabetic benefits of turmeric and curcumin occur because of a number of other specific actions that they perform on various interrelated, common factors known to cause and exacerbate type II diabetes and pre-diabetes. These actions include:

- hindering insulin resistance.

- improving abnormalities in cholesterol metabolism associated with diabetes.

- lowering levels of free fatty acids and hemoglobin A1c.

- reducing blood glucose (sugar) levels.

- slowing the production of glucose by the liver.

Studies have also shown that turmeric and curcumin not only help to minimize the above factors, but that they also are capable of stimulating insulin production in the pancreas and also improving the activity of pancreas cells. Both turmeric and curcumin have even been shown to help repair and regenerate pancreas cells. Moreover, studies also show that they can improve the ability of the body to most efficiently make use of glucose.

Treating Diabetes Symptoms

Just as significantly, research has also confirmed that turmeric and curcumin provide effective benefits as natural treatments for serious symptoms caused by type II diabetes, including:

- improving and enhancing impaired wound healing.

- preventing and reversing gastroparesis, a common gastrointestinal condition affecting diabetes patients that is characterized by a delay in the movement of the food from stomach into the intestines, leading to spikes in glucose levels.

- stopping bone loss associated with diabetes.

- preventing and improving the symptoms of vision disorders caused by diabetes, including retinopathy.

- protecting against cardiovascular conditions that diabetic and pre-diabetic patients are at greater risk of developing.

- shielding kidneys from damage caused by diabetic neuropathy.

- providing pain relief caused by diabetic neuropathy.

- reversing fatty liver disease, which is common in diabetic patients.

Studies on the Benefits of Turmeric and Curcumin for Type II Diabetes

Let's take a closer look at what some of the many research studies conducted on the subject have found about turmeric's and curcumin's benefits for preventing and treating pre- and type II diabetes. As mentioned, diabetes is an inflammatory condition. Research has shown that turmeric and curcumin can reduce various proteins, enzymes, and other compounds that are known to be factors in type II diabetes, thus reducing inflammation in people suffering from the disease.

Reducing Inflammation

One such study involved 100 hundred patients diagnosed with type II diabetes. It was conducted over a three-month period, and demonstrated some of the potential ways for which turmeric and curcumin provide anti-diabetic benefits.

In this study, the patients were divided into two groups, with fifty participants in each group. At the beginning of the study, all the participants in each group were tested to measure their levels of serum adipocyte-fatty acid binding protein (A-FABP) levels. The A-FABP protein is known to negatively impact metabolism when its levels are elevated in the body. Also measured were the patient's levels of C-reactive protein (CRP), tumor necrosis factor-α, and interleukin-6, all of which are markers of chronic inflammation in the body that can worsen diabetes' symptoms. The patients' glucose and free fatty acid (FFA) levels were also assessed, as was the amount and activity of superoxide dismutase (SOD), one of the body's most powerful antioxidant enzymes.

Throughout the study, one of the groups acted as the placebo group, while the other fifty participants were given turmeric extracts (curcuminoids) on a daily basis. By the end of the study, its researchers found that the turmeric extracts resulted in "significant decreases in serum A-FABP, C-reactive protein (CRP), tumor necrosis factor-α, and interleukin-6 levels." The turmeric extracts also "significantly increased serum superoxide dismutase (SOD) activity."

The study's researchers noted that "[t]he change in serum A-FABP levels showed positive correlations with changes in levels of glucose, free fatty acids (FFAs), and CRP in subjects supplemented with curcuminoids. Further stepwise regression analysis showed that A-FABP was an independent predictor for levels of FFAs, SOD, and CRP. These results suggest that curcuminoids may exert anti-diabetic effects, at least in part, by reductions in serum A-FABP level. A-FABP reduction is associated with improved metabolic parameters in human Type II diabetes." These findings prove that turmeric extracts can help reduce inflammation in cases of type II diabetes.

Reduction of Oxidative Stress and Risk of Heart Disease

Other studies have also demonstrated that curcuminoids from turmeric can also help reduce oxidative stress in type II diabetes patients. One such study also found that curcuminoids not only reduce oxidative stress, but also reduce the risk of heart disease associated with type II diabetes to a similar degree as statin drugs. This is vitally important information for type II diabetes patients to know, since statin drugs can cause a variety of harmful side effects, whereas no such side effects are caused by turmeric or its extracts, even when taken in high doses.

This particular study examined the effects on a specific type of turmeric extract, compared to a statin drug, on the endothelial function of type II diabetes patients. Endothelial cells make up the lining of blood and lymph vessels known as the *endothelium*. Dysfunction of the endothelium can cause endothelial cells to become over-activated which, as you learned in Chapter 5, can result in the buildup of vulnerable plaque in the arteries, a primary risk factor for heart attack, stroke, and other forms of heart disease. Endothelial dysfunction is often present in type II diabetes patients at risk for heart disease.

The study began with seventy-two patients with type II diabetes, sixty-seven of whom completed it after eight weeks. Researchers compared the effects of NCB-02 (a standardized preparation of curcuminoids) to the statin drug atorvastatin (Lipitor) on the patients' endothelial function and associated biomarkers. The endothelial function of all of the patients was measured at the beginning of the study. Blood samples were also collected at the beginning of the study to measure the patients' levels of malondialdehyde (a compound in the body that is a marker for oxidative stress), an indicator of endothelial function called endothelin-1 (ET-1), and two markers for inflammation and oxidative stress, interleukin-6 (IL-6) and tumour necrosis factor-alpha (TNF-alpha). According to the researchers who conducted this study, at its beginning "there was no significant difference in the various parameters tested" among any of the patients, and all of the patients were found to have a similar degree of endothelial dysfunction.

The patients were then randomly divided into three groups. The first group was given a placebo, the second group received atorvastatin (10 mg once a day), and the third group received NCB-02 (two capsules containing 150 mg of curcumin taken twice a day).

At the end of the study, all of the above measurements were again taken and compared to the initial findings. There were no changes in the placebo group, but both the atorvastatin and NCB-02 groups both achieved comparable "significant improvement" in their endothelial function. "Similarly," the researchers wrote, "patients receiving atorvastatin or NCB-02 showed significant reductions in the levels of malondialdehyde, ET-1, IL-6 and TNF-alpha," concluding that "NCB-02 had a favorable effect, comparable to that of atorvastatin, on endothelial dysfunction in association with reductions in inflammatory cytokines and markers of oxidative stress."

Lessening of Blood Sugar Levels and Restraint of Insulin Resistance

Research has also shown that both turmeric and curcumin have a direct effect on blood sugar and insulin levels, with both substances having been proven to be able to lower blood sugar and help prevent insulin resistance. These facts were clearly demonstrated in a scientific review and analysis of studies on turmeric and curcumin published in the medical database PubMed between 1998 and 2013.

This analysis revealed that turmeric and curcumin can reverse the "many pathophysiological processes involved in development and progression of hyperglycemia [high blood sugar] and insulin resistance." Specifically, the authors of the analysis found that, "Curcumin can reduce blood glucose level by reducing the hepatic glucose production, suppression of hyperglycemia-induced inflammatory state, stimulation of glucose uptake by up-regulation of GLUT4, GLUT2 and GLUT3 genes expressions, activation of AMP kinase, promoting the PPAR ligand-binding activity, stimulation of insulin secretion from pancreatic tissues, improvement in pancreatic cell function, and reduction of insulin resistance."

A more recent study also confirmed curcumin's benefits in improving blood sugar levels in type II diabetes patients, as well as in lowering their LDL ("bad") cholesterol levels and body mass index (BMI), and in improving their overall lipid profiles. The study involved seventy patients with type II diabetes, who randomly divided into two groups in a three-month-long double-blind clinical trial. There were no significant differences in the mean age, sex, BMI, fasting blood glucose levels, total cholesterol levels, HDL and

LDL cholesterol, triglycerides, or hemoglobin A1c (HbA1c) levels between the patients in both groups, all of which were measured at the beginning of the study and at its conclusion.

One group of patients in the study received a daily dose of 80 mg of a specific type of curcumin supplement (nano-micelle curcumin, a form that significantly improves curcumin's absorption rate in the body), while the other group received a placebo each day. By the study's end, compared to the placebo group, the curcumin group exhibited "a significant decrease" in their fasting blood glucose, triglyceride, and HbA1C levels, as well as in their body mass index. The LDL levels were also found to have decreased.

Prevention of Type II Diabetes

The above studies are only a sampling of the many clinical trials that have been conducted on turmeric and curcumin which confirm the many important benefits they can offer to people suffering from type II diabetes. But perhaps the most important benefit they provide is their ability to prevent type II diabetes in the first place, even in people who are at high risk for developing this all too prevalent disease. This is especially true of curcumin, as an important study published in *Diabetes Care,* the medical journal published by the American Diabetes Association, proved.

This study was a randomized, double-blind, placebo-controlled trial that involved 240 participants above the age of thirty-five, all of whom met the American Diabetes Association's criteria for having pre-diabetes. The aim of the study, its researchers wrote, was to determine whether or not curcumin is effective for delaying the onset of type II diabetes in people with pre-diabetes.

The study ran for a period of nine months. For three months prior to its beginning, all the selected participants were educated on the importance of a healthy lifestyle, with an emphasis on a standardized healthy diet and a recommended program of regular exercise. They were shown how to follow such a diet and incorporate the recommended exercises into their daily lives and asked to do so for the duration of the study itself. The participants were then randomly assigned to two groups. The first group received three placebo capsules taken orally twice a day, and the second group received three capsules of curcumin at a dose of 250 mg that were also taken orally twice a day.

At its start, then again at three and six months, and finally at the end of the study, all of the participants were tested by the researchers to assess if their condition was progressing to type II diabetes. This was done by looking for changes in their beta cells' functioning, using what is known as a homeostasis model assessment [HOMA]-β, in conjunction with monitoring the participants' C-peptide levels and activity, and their beta-cells' proinsulin/insulin ratio. Also monitored and evaluated were their body weight, their waist circumference to measure their degree of abdominal obesity, their level of insulin resistance, and their level of the anti-inflammatory cytokine adiponectin. The subjects in the curcumin group were also tested to determine whether curcumin caused them any adverse effects.

By the sixth month of the study, eleven members of the placebo group (9.5 percent) developed type II diabetes. By the study's end, this number rose to nineteen, or 16.4 percent of the group's participants. Throughout the study, no one in the curcumin group developed type II diabetes. Instead, their health measurements began to show improvements by month six that had increased by the study's end. As the researchers wrote, "HOMA-β in the curcumin-treated group was increasingly elevated in all follow-up visits (at three, six, and nine months) and became statistically significant at the final visit (nine months). Blood levels of C-peptide were found to be significantly lower in curcumin-treated group when compared with those of placebo group. Although not significant, proinsulin/insulin ratio showed a lower trend in the curcumin-treated group."

In addition, within the curcumin group, researchers found that their levels of insulin resistance was lower compared to the placebo group beginning at three months. The researchers observed that:

> The differences were significant, particularly at the six and nine month visits. Levels of adiponectin, an anti-inflammatory cytokine, in the placebo-treated group were virtually unchanged, whereas those of the curcumin-treated group were gradually elevated (at three and six months) and became significantly different from that of placebo-treated group at the final visit (nine months).

They also reported that some of the participants in the curcumin group also lost weight and reduced their waist size. Moreover, throughout the study, curcumin caused no incidence of adverse effects. At the conclusion of their published study, the researchers wrote, "Because of its benefits and safety, we propose that curcumin extract may be used for an intervention therapy for the prediabetic population."

The findings of this study are important. As Benjamin Franklin noted centuries ago, "An ounce of prevention is worth a pound of cure." According to the Centers for Disease Control and Prevention (CDC), today in the United States, over 84 million Americans over the age of eighteen already suffer from pre-diabetes. Unless it is properly addressed, pre-diabetes will not only inevitably develop into type II diabetes, it also dramatically increases the likelihood of the life-threatening diseases type II diabetes has been linked to, such as heart disease, stroke, cancer, and Alzheimer's disease. Yet we now have scientific evidence that this unhealthy trend can, in large part, be prevented simply by adding a curcumin supplement to our daily routine. The potential curcumin has in this regard cannot be overemphasized.

Curcumin May Offer Benefits for Type I Diabetes

Unlike type II diabetes, which, in many cases, can be completely cured with the proper combination of lifestyle changes, including regular exercise, weight loss, diet, and the use of turmeric, curcumin, and other nutritional supplements, Type I diabetes is considered incurable. It is an autoimmune condition caused by the infiltration of white blood cells known as lymphocyte, as well as the destruction of beta cells (β-cells) within the islets of Langerhans, the part of the pancreas that produces insulin and other hormones. In type I diabetes, the pancreas's β-cells decline in both their numbers and volume, causing severe and permanent insulin deficiency. Because of this, people with type I diabetes are dependent on daily insulin injections or the use of insulin pumps.

A preliminary animal study published in the medical journal *Diabetology & Metabolic Syndrome* indicates that curcumin may offer hope for type I diabetic patients, not as a cure, but as a significant aid for helping to reverse various important factors associated with the disease. In the study, researchers induced type I diabetes in rats. The rats were then divided into two groups, with the first group acting as the control. The rats in the second group were given an oral "novel curcumin derivative" (NCD) once a day for forty days.

Both groups of rats were then observed and tested for a period of ten months. Fasting blood samples were taken from both groups throughout the length of the study to measure the rats' plasma glucose, insulin and C-peptide levels. In addition, tissue samples were also taken and examined using microscopes in order to assess the condition of the rats' pancreatic islets as the study progressed. Aside from the NCD supplement, both groups of rats followed the same diet throughout the study.

Ending this section with this conclusion reached by the authors of a published meta-analysis entitled *Curcumin and Diabetes: A Systematic Review* seems most apt. They wrote:

Recent research has provided the scientific basis for "traditional" curcumin and confirmed the important role of curcumin in the prevention and treatment of diabetes and its associated disorders. Curcumin could

---

For the first four months, neither group of rats showed changes in their glucose, insulin, and C-peptide levels. By the fourth month, however, the NCD group began to exhibit a gradual decrease in their glucose levels and increases in their insulin and C-peptide levels. By the end of the study (ten months), these levels were almost normal and on par with those of healthy, non-diabetic rats. As the researchers wrote, "NCD treated diabetic rats showed significantly lowered plasma glucose and increased plasma insulin and C-peptide levels. This was followed by a further significant decrease in plasma glucose and [an] increase in plasma insulin and C-peptide after two months from oral administration of the NCD. The plasma insulin and C-peptide continued to increase for ten months reaching levels significantly higher than the basal [starting point] level."

Even more significantly, after six months, the pancreases of the NCD-treated rats "showed the appearance of small, well-formed islets and positive insulin cells," and by ten months the pancreases of the NCD rat group "showed well-developed, larger sized islets with disappearance of primitive cell collections ad CD 105 positive cells. Also, insulin positive islets of variable size with disappearance of insulin positive cells in adipose tissue were detected." What this means is that the curcumin derivative was shown to repair and regenerate the islets.

The researchers concluded their study by writing, "Our current data suggest that the NCD can significantly ameliorate [improve] experimental Type I diabetes. Our study provides clear evidence of pancreatic islets regeneration in response to treatment of diabetic rats with the NCD for forty days. This could be attributed to the anti-inflammatory and antioxidant effects of curcumin and thus creates a favorable systemic and pancreatic environment to foster islet neogenesis [regeneration]. Also, the role of curcumin in cell proliferation and differentiation of stem cells may be involved." Hopefully, one day the mechanisms of action of this curcumin derivative will lead to similar benefits to humans suffering from type I diabetes.

favorably affect most of the leading aspects of diabetes, including insulin resistance, hyperglycemia, hyperlipidemia, and islet apoptosis and necrosis. In addition, curcimin could prevent the deleterious [harmful] complications of diabetes. Despite the potential tremendous benefits of this multifaceted nature product, results from clinical trials of curcumin are only available in using curcumin to treat diabetic nephropathy, microangiopathy and retinopathy so far.

Studies are badly needed to be done in humans to confirm the potential of curcumin in limitation of diabetes and other associated disorders. Further, multiple approaches are also needed to overcome limited solubility and poor bioavailability of curcumin. These include synthesis of curcuminoids and development of novel formulations of curcumin, such as nanoparticles, liposomal encapsulation, emulsions, and sustained released tablets. Enhanced bioavailability and convinced clinical trial results of curcumin are likely to bring this promising natural product to the forefront of therapeutic agents for diabetes by generating a "super curcumin" in the near future.

I have no doubt that their prediction will prove to be correct. Yet, I don't recommend that you wait for such a "super curcumin" product to appear. Instead, get started right now putting curcumin and turmeric to work for you using the high quality products that are already available.

OTHER STEPS YOU CAN TAKE TO PREVENT AND MANAGE DIABETES

Once again, in spite of all the important benefits turmeric and curcumin provide for preventing and helping reverse and relief the symptoms of diabetes, they are not "magic bullet" solutions for the disease. Rather, a multi-pronged overall lifestyle approach is necessary. The two most important elements to such an approach are adopting a healthy diet and getting regular exercise.

Diet

Unlike type I diabetes, type II diabetes and pre-diabetes are primarily due to poor lifestyle choices. This is especially true of poor dietary choices.

One of the most important dietary steps you need to take is to eliminate all refined sugars and sugar products from your diet. Common dietary sources of sugar include:

- corn syrup and sweeteners
- cornstarch
- dextrin
- dextrose
- fructose

- fruit juice concentrates
- glucose
- lactose

- malt
- maltodextrin
- maltose
- mannitol

- sorbitol
- sorghum
- sucrose
- xylitol

Also avoid all so-called fast, or junk, foods, soda, and other sweetened beverages, including many commercial fruit juices. Reducing or eliminating your intake of alcohol is also recommended.

To further help better regulate your body's blood glucose levels, also limit your overall carbohydrate intake and replace simple carbohydrates with complex carbohydrate foods, such as whole grains, beans, legumes, and other fiber-rich vegetables. Eating protein-rich foods as snacks between meals can also help.

A healthy dietary anti-diabetes approach is to eat according to the glycemic index. This means eating foods that have negligible impact on blood sugar and insulin levels when they are consumed. Foods that have a high glycemic rating cause the greatest spikes in blood sugar and insulin levels, while foods with a low glycemic index have a minimal impacts. Low-glycemic foods include raw, organic leafy green vegetables, fruits that contain pits, sweet potatoes, yams, most legumes and nuts, skim milk and buttermilk, poultry, white fish, shellfish, and lean cuts of beef and veal.

Foods with a high-glycemic rating include white breads, bagels, English muffins, commercially packaged cereals, cookies, pastries, and most other desserts, raisins and dried fruits, whole milk and cheeses (both of which are high in lactose, a type of sugar), peanuts, peanut butter, hot dogs, and luncheon meats. Such foods are best avoided altogether.

Exercise

Regular exercise and physical activity is the other primary aspect, along with a healthy diet, that is necessary for preventing and reversing pre- and type II diabetes. To be effective, you do not need to engage in strenuous exercise. In fact, research shows that strenuous exercise can be counterproductive because of how it can trigger and perpetuate inflammation in the body. Light exercise is a much better choice. This can include walking, swimming, bicycling, and any other types of exercise that cause you to sweat and temporarily increase your heart rate. Regularly engaging in light exercise for thirty to sixty minutes a day not only helps to control unhealthy weight gain, but also lowers and helps regulate blood sugar and insulin levels.

In addition to the proper diet and regular exercise, schedule regular annual testing with your physician to screen for early signs of blood sugar problems. Also, become proactive and learn what works best for you in terms of managing your blood sugar and other metabolic factors. Get tested to screen for food allergies and sensitivities that may also be predisposing you towards developing diabetes. Such foods can impair, and even destroy, pancreas cells in your body due to the autoimmune reactions they cause.

Certain other nutritional supplements can also be helpful when taken in conjunction with turmeric and curcumin. These include B vitamins, vitamin C, vitamin E, coenzyme Q_{10} (CoQ_{10}), chromium, magnesium, potassium, and zinc.

Finally, do your best to manage stress in your life, because stress is a major cause of chronic inflammation and can also increase blood sugar and insulin levels.

CONCLUSION

I hope that by reading this chapter, you are now motivated to make a high quality curcumin product part of your daily health routine, and that you will also start using turmeric more frequently as a spice for your meals. By doing so, you will be protecting yourself from the scourges of both pre- and type II diabetes. In the process, you will also be lowering your risk of the many other health conditions these diseases are known to cause.

Now let's turn our attention to even more health problems that turmeric and curcumin can help you avoid or reverse. That is the topic of the next chapter.

9

Other Health Benefits of Turmeric & Curcumin

I n the previous chapters of this book, you learned about the main health conditions for which both turmeric and curcumin have been shown by scientific research to offer significant benefits. You also learned that it is their anti-inflammatory and antioxidant properties that are the main reasons they can be so effective in preventing and helping to reverse those conditions.

In this chapter, you will learn about various other health conditions for which turmeric and curcumin can be helpful. Let's begin by first exploring some other important health-promoting properties turmeric and curcumin possess for helping to protect against infectious microorganisms.

BOOSTING IMMUNITY

Research has confirmed that, in addition to their anti-inflammatory and antioxidant properties, turmeric and curcumin can help boost and maintain immune function because of the protection they offer against harmful infections. Specifically, both substances have been shown to protect against infections from bacteria and viruses.

Bacteria

As you learned in Chapter 6, studies have shown that turmeric and curcumin are effective in combating *Heliobacter pylori* (H. pylori), a type of bacteria that is known to cause both gastric and peptic ulcers and other gastrointestinal conditions, as well as stomach cancer, internal bleeding, and anemia, among other health problems. As you also learned in Chapter 6, turmeric and curcumin are effective natural treatments for H. pylori because of their ability to block the bacteria's growth and spread within the stomach, in part by destroying the protective coating of biofilm that can otherwise prevent the body's immune system from detecting and eliminating it.

Other studies have shown that turmeric and curcumin also protect against other harmful bacteria, including *streptococcus* and *staphylococcus*. Streptococcus bacteria, or "strep," are most known for causing strep throat, but they can also cause a number of other diseases, some of them quite serious, such as scarlet fever and toxic shock syndrome. Strep is also a cause of the infectious skin condition impetigo. The most virulent strains of streptococcus can also cause necrotizing fasciitis, which is more commonly known as flesh-eating disease. Other strains of strep can cause blood infections, pneumonia, and meningitis (especially in infants).

Staphylococcus, or "staph" bacteria most often cause a variety of skin conditions, but they too can also cause blood infection, pneumonia, and toxic shock syndrome. Staph bacteria are also a common cause of food poisoning.

Like H. pylori, both strep and staph bacteria can elude the body's immune system because of biofilm coatings that hide them from immune cells. Turmeric and curcumin can help destroy these coatings just as they do H. pylori's biofilm. One study, for example, found that turmeric extract can inhibit the formation and growth of strep biofilm by over 78 percent. Other research has shown similar results when turmeric extracts come in contact with staph bacteria.

Viruses

Research has also shown that turmeric and curcumin act as potent, natural antiviral agents, including offering protection against the most common cause of viral infections in humans, the Epstein Barr virus (EBV). EBV is a strain within the family of human herpes viruses and is also known as human herpes virus—4, or HHV—4. It affects virtually all of us at some point in our lives, yet in many cases does so without causing any symptoms. However, when the body's immune system becomes compromised, EBV can cause a variety of disease conditions, ranging from cold and flu, to mononucleosis, which in some cases can be life-threatening.

EBV is also a common factor in chronic fatigue syndrome (CFS), especially cases in which fatigue and CFS's related symptoms are crippling in severity. EBV can also be a contributing factor in multiple sclerosis (MS), and has also been linked to different types of cancer, including Burkitt's lymphoma, Hodgkin's disease, and non-Hodgkin's lymphoma. It can be a co-factor in AIDS, as well. Currently, conventional medicine has no known cure for EBV.

Like all other types of viruses, EBV harms the body and causes disease by inserting itself into cells. Once this invasion takes hold, EBV is then able to spread to and invade other cells. Research has found that turmeric, and especially curcumin, can effectively halt this spread of EBV in the body by inhibiting various protein compounds within EBV that cause the virus to be activated and become more dangerous.

Both turmeric and curcumin also provide significant protection against flu viruses. Research shows that curcumin in particular is capable of reducing the replication of flu viruses in human cells by more than 90 percent. Other research found that an oral spray of turmeric oil is also effective for inhibiting various flu viruses. Clinical studies have also shown that both turmeric and curcumin help reduce flu-related coughs, fever, and mucus buildup in the lungs.

Curcumin has also been shown to protect against HIV (human immunodeficiency virus). As with EBV, its protective actions against HIV have to do with its ability to inhibit components with the virus that are necessary for it to replicate (grow and spread). In fact, curcumin's anti-HIV properties are so impressive that some researchers wrote, "[C]urcumin and its analogues may have the potential for novel drug development against HIV."

Other illnesses that turmeric and curcumin can help protect against and inhibit the spread of include adenoviruses, which cause upper respiratory conditions; hepatitis C, a virus that attacks and causes inflammation to the liver and can lead to hepatitis; cirrhosis, or chronic liver damage; and liver cancer.

In addition to the antibacterial and antiviral properties turmeric and curcumin possess, additional research has also shown that both natural substances can further protect the immune system because they are effective in combating various types of fungus, as well as infectious protozoa (single-cell parasites such as giardia).

AIDING DETOXIFICATION
AND PREVENTING IRON OVERLOAD

Another important health benefit that turmeric and curcumin provide has to do with their roles as natural detoxification agents. As you learned earlier in this book, turmeric and curcumin have both been shown by scientific research to protect and enhance the functioning of the kidneys, gallbladder, and liver, all of which play crucially important roles in helping to carry out your body's detoxification processes. By helping to keep these organs healthy, turmeric and curcumin enhance their ability to help your body detoxify.

This is particularly true of the health-promoting benefits they provide to the liver. That's because, when it comes to detoxification, your liver, of all internal organs in your body, is the most important, carrying out numerous detoxification processes in addition to the literally hundreds of other tasks it is responsible for on a moment-by-moment basis.

All of us are exposed to thousands of different types of toxins on a daily basis. They exist within our air, soil, and water supplies, in the foods and water we drink, and in many home and household products, including furniture and even children's toys. When the body's ability to detoxify itself from this toxic onslaught becomes impaired for any length of time, disease inevitably follows, including life-threatening illness such as Alzheimer's disease, cancer, heart attack, and stroke. The buildup of toxins in the body is also one of the primary causes of premature aging.

Among the most pernicious types of disease-causing toxins are heavy metals, especially aluminum, arsenic, cadmium, fluoride, lead, and mercury, exposures to which today are much higher than they were even a few short decades ago. But even the body's own supply of naturally occurring metals, such as copper, iron, and zinc, can also be problematic. This is especially true of iron.

What Is Iron Overload?

We all need iron in order to stay healthy and have more energy. However, when the body's iron stores become excessive, a condition known as iron overload (or *hemochromatosis*), when iron overload becomes especially severe, our health can become compromised due to the toxic buildup of heavy metals from the environment. As we age, iron levels in our bodies naturally begin to increase within cells and tissues. Excess iron levels, however, are known to damage mitochondria (the cells' "energy factories") and can become major contributors of free radical damage to cells, tissues, and organs.

Even more alarming, scientists have confirmed that iron overload is a significant factor that can cause liver damage and liver disease, such as liver fibrosis, and plays a major role in increasing the risk of cancer, heart disease, Alzheimer's disease and dementia, and Parkinson's disease. Because of these facts, scientists and health experts alike now point out that limiting the buildup of iron in our bodies is an important step towards reducing the risk of developing such diseases. As it turns out, recent research has found that the use of turmeric and curcumin is an effective means of achieving this goal.

Numerous studies in recent years have demonstrated that both turmeric and curcumin act as potent natural iron chelators, meaning that they both possess the ability to directly move excess iron out of cells and tissues so they can then be eliminated through the body's various detoxification pathways. But that is not the only benefit that turmeric and curcumin provide for preventing and reversing iron overload. Researchers have also found that both substances, especially curcumin, increase the genetic expression of ferritin, a transport protein in the body that binds iron, keeping it away from vulnerable cells and tissues. Moreover, research has also shown that turmeric's and curcumin's ability to chelate iron help to protect and restore the body's DNA repair mechanisms. This, in turn, helps to prevent neurons in the brain from becoming damaged by iron overload and other toxic exposures, thus reducing the risk of neurodegenerative conditions such as Alzheimer's and Parkinson's disease.

Finally, the discovery of iron-chelating properties of turmeric and curcumin further explains why both substances are so effective for helping the body's immune system defend itself from harmful, infectious microorganisms. That's because many of these microorganisms need to bind with iron in the body in order to thrive and spread.

As you learned in Chapter 3, turmeric and curcumin have also been shown to be effective for preventing and removing the buildup of fluoride in the body. Additional research has also confirmed that turmeric and curcumin confer the same types of benefits for protecting against other heavy metals, as well, including arsenic, cadmium, lead, and mercury. Given all of these facts, turmeric and curcumin are clearly important natural aids you can use to better protect yourself from such dangerous toxins. Now let's take a look at some of the other health conditions for which turmeric and curcumin can be beneficial.

EYE CONDITIONS

Many vision problems are caused by a combination of chronic inflammation and free radical damage caused by oxidation. Because of its anti-inflammatory and antioxidant properties, curcumin has been shown by researchers to have potential benefits for eye conditions, including cataracts, dry eye, glaucoma, age-related macular degeneration, and other vision disorders.

Curcumin's neuroprotective properties also play a significant role in the way that it can protect eye health. That's because the retina of the eye originates as an outgrowth of the brain during fetal development and is considered part of the central nervous system. Like the brain, the retina also contains various types of neuronal cells. In Chapter 3, you learned how curcumin is able to protect brain neurons and thus help to maintain brain health. In much the same way, it is able to protect retinal health, as well.

Given all of these benefits that it provides, researchers have studied its potential benefits for retinal eye diseases and other eye problems for over two decades. Based on their findings, they have described curcumin as "a potent, therapeutic drug candidate for inflammatory and degenerative retinal and eye diseases." And in addition to recommending curcumin supplements to help protect eye health, today scientists are also exploring the use of curcumin in eye drops.

Additional research has been conducted on curcumin's potential benefits for protecting the cornea of the eye, and thus as an aid for problems known as *anterior segment eye diseases,* including cataracts, conjunctivitis, and glaucoma, which are often related to inflammation and oxidative stress. Thus far, laboratory and animal studies have shown that curcumin can help prevent corneal eye conditions by impeding inflammation in the eyes, inhibiting the activity of cytokines known to cause eye disease.

Curcumin also protects the cornea from bacterial infections, helping to repair corneal wound healing and preventing free radical damage, including preventing lipid peroxidation (free radical damage to the lipid, or fat, structures in the eyes). It prevents changes and degradation of proteins in the lenses of the eyes. It also defends against angiogenesis, which is a major factor in the development of *corneal NV,* a condition in which excessive blood vessels grow into the cornea. Corneal NV is the leading cause of blindness in the United States.

All of these eye-healing properties of curcumin have led researchers to conclude that "curcumin's harmless nature, low cost, and multiple targeting potential make it a promising agent for the prevention and treatment of various eye diseases. Accumulating evidence has demonstrated its potential therapeutic value."

MULTIPLE SCLEROSIS

Multiple sclerosis, or MS, is an autoimmune condition that affects the central nervous system. In cases of MS, the immune system becomes overactivated and begins to attack and remove sections of the protective and insulating covering of nerve fibers, causing the nerve fibers themselves to become scarred and hardened. This covering is known as the *myelin sheath.*

Damage to the myelin sheath impairs nerve transmission from the brain to the muscles and other parts of the body, leading to numerous symptoms that range from muscle pain, chronic fatigue, numbness and pain in the feet and hands, balance and walking problems, sensitivity to heat and cold, and vision problems. In some cases, MS can also cause severe weakness or partial or complete paralysis, making patients wheelchair-bound. Another troubling aspect of MS is that its symptoms are usually intermittent, meaning they can flare up and then go into remission, only to strike without warning later, usually more severely.

Research has shown that turmeric and curcumin can help lessen symptoms of MS. Both substances are able to do so for the same reasons that they have proven so effective as natural aids for other autoimmune conditions such as rheumatoid arthritis (see Chapter 7) and inflammatory bowel disease (see Chapter 6). Specifically, they regulate the body's pro-inflammatory cytokines, as well as the NF-kappaB signaling pathways in immune cells. By doing so, they help to reduce levels of chronic inflammation, a primary trigger for MS. In addition, as you've learned throughout this book, turmeric and curcumin are potent antioxidants. Because of this, they are able to reduce oxidation and the free radical damage it causes, both of which play major roles in the development of MS and the flare ups of its many symptoms.

Research has shown that the neuroprotective benefits turmeric and curcumin provide, which you learned about in Chapter 3, are also very helpful in helping to relieve MS symptoms. Some researchers have described MS as "a coordinated immune attack across the blood brain barrier." As Chapter 3 revealed, turmeric is one of very few natural substances that is capable of crossing the blood brain barrier, where it goes to work nourishing and protecting the brain's neurons, nerve fibers, and neuronal pathways.

All told, while turmeric and curcumin are certainly not cures for MS, they should definitely be considered effective natural remedies for helping to manage the symptoms of this difficult-to-treat disease.

PARKINSON'S DISEASE

Because both turmeric and curcumin provide neuroprotective benefits, they hold promise as natural aids in treating Parkinson's disease. This is particularly true of curcumin.

Research has revealed that the development of Parkinson's disease, a progressive degenerative condition for which there currently is no cure, begins with the aggregation, or clumping together, of a class of proteins known as *alpha-synuclein proteins* with other proteins in the body. Scientists at Michigan State University (MSU) have discovered that curcumin helps to prevent this process from occurring.

"Our research shows that curcumin can rescue proteins from aggregation, the first steps of many debilitating diseases," said Lisa Lapidus, an MSU associate professor who co-authored a published study of these findings. "More specifically, curcumin binds strongly to alpha-synuclein and prevents aggregation at body temperatures."

Lapidus and her colleagues used lasers to study protein folding, the process by which proteins are built from chains of amino acids. The research conducted by Lapidus and her team helped to shed light on this protein folding process "by correlating the speed at which protein folds with its tendency to clump or bind with other proteins." As they conducted their research, they discovered that curcumin is able to bind to alpha-synuclein proteins. As it does so, it not only stops the proteins from clumping together, it also increases the protein's folding rate. By doing so, it also prevents alpha-synuclein proteins from clumping with other proteins.

Other research has shown that curcumin offers other potential benefits as a treatment for Parkinson's disease that current pharmaceutical drugs do not provide. Such drugs are primarily focused on replenishing dopamine levels in the brain. Although they can help to relieve symptoms in the early stages of Parkinson's disease, they do not prevent the progression of the disease itself, and over time they often result in balance problems and difficulties walking. Moreover, as researchers noted in the medical journal *Current Pharmaceutical Design,* most drugs used to treat Parkinson's disease "do not exhibit neuroprotective effects in patients," whereas curcumin does provide important neuroprotective benefits.

Research also shows that curcumin demonstrated neuroprotective properties in an animal model of Parkinson's disease. According to researchers, this beneficial effect is related, in part, to curcumin's antioxidant properties and its ability to cross the blood brain barrier and reach neurons and other brain cells.

In addition, curcumin counteracts the effects of glutathione depletion in the body. Glutathione is one of the body's most important compounds that protects against free radical damage. Its depletion in the body causes oxidative stress, impaired mitochondria function, and premature cell death. Lack of glutathione is known to be a factor in the onset of early Parkinson's disease.

Curcumin's neuroprotective benefits for Parkinson's disease are due in part to its ability to inhibit what is known as the *c-Jun N-terminal kinase* (JNK) signaling pathway. This pathway is involved in the death and degeneration of dopamine-containing (dopaminergic) neurons, which is known to be another causative factor of Parkinson's disease. Therefore, curcumin's ability to prevent dopaminergic neuronal death inhibiting the JNK pathway is significant. All of these findings explain why researchers continue to study curcumin as they seek to better understand and treat Parkinson's disease.

PREMENSTRUAL SYNDROME (PMS)

PMS affects nearly all women at some time in their lives, causing symptoms such as bloating, cramps, and pain, as well as moodiness and other emotional issues in the days leading up to menstruation. Researchers have found that curcumin can effectively relieve such PMS symptoms.

In one clinical, double-blind study, women who regularly suffered from PMS were randomly divided into two groups. Before the study began, all of the women were evaluated for the severity and range of PMS symptoms they experienced. The evaluation examined three categories of symptoms: psychological symptoms, such as feelings of irritability, anxiety, depression or sadness, crying, or feelings of isolation; physical symptoms, such as abdominal pain, backache, headache, breast tenderness, weight gain, bloating, muscle stiffness, gastrointestinal symptoms, or nausea; and behavioral symptoms, such as fatigue, insomnia, difficulty concentrating, or changes in appetite. There was no statistical difference in any of these categories between the women in both groups.

The study ran for three menstrual cycles. For seven days prior to, and three days after each cycle, the first group of women were given two placebo capsules and asked to keep a record of their symptoms and their severity using a daily questionnaire. The women in the second group received two capsules of curcumin during the same time frames, and were also asked to record their answers on the daily questionnaire. By the study's conclusion, the women in the curcumin group showed significant reductions in their symptoms across all three categories, while the placebo group showed no significant improvement. The authors of the study wrote, "Our results for the first time showed a potential advantageous effect of curcumin in attenuating severity of PMS symptoms, which were probably mediated by modulation of neurotransmitters and anti-inflammatory effects of curcumin."

PSORIASIS

Psoriasis is a skin condition that usually affects the outside of the knees, elbows, scalp, or lower back. It is characterized by thick, reddish patching of the skin. The patches may sometimes also be covered by silvery scales. Unlike other skin conditions, psoriasis typically does not cause itching.

Chronic inflammation is a significant cause of psoriasis, especially inflammation triggered by the pro-inflammatory cytokines known as *tumor necrosis factors* (TNFs), particularly tumor necrosis factor-alpha (TNF-α), which you first learned about in Chapter 2. For this reason, TNF-blocking drugs are typically prescribed by dermatologists and other physicians as a treatment for psoriasis. Ultraviolet (UV) light therapies are also sometimes used.

As you also learned earlier in this book, curcumin is a significant natural aid for inhibiting over-activity of TNF-α in the body. As a result, its potential for helping to prevent and heal psoriasis have been explored by researchers for a number of years, and the findings are quite promising.

According to researchers, curcumin can benefit psoriasis sufferers in a number of ways, starting with its proven ability to inhibit and block the production of TNF-α as well as inhibiting the activity of other pro-inflammatory compounds in skin cells that are induced by TNF-signaling. In addition, curcumin has been shown to be toxic to infectious agents associated with psoriasis, such as *E. coli* and *Salmonella typhimurium*, even in very low doses. Curcumin also has shown promise for potentially enhancing the effectiveness of UV light therapy for psoriasis.

In addition to TNF-α, another compound that is known to be involved in the development of psoriasis is *phosphorylase kinase* (PhK). Elevated levels of PhK are associated with the skin condition, and curcumin has been shown to be a potent inhibitor of PhK activity. In one study, a gel containing only one percent curcumin was found to significantly decrease PhK activity. In another study, daily oral supplementation of a curcumin capsule (4,500 mg per dose) was found to reduce psoriasis symptoms by as much as 88 percent within twelve weeks.

WEIGHT LOSS

In Chapter 2 of this book, you learned that chronic inflammation is a causative factor in unhealthy weight gain and obesity, and that it also makes losing weight more difficult. Chronic inflammation and being unhealthily overweight or obese can combine to create a vicious cycle, with chronic inflammation triggering and perpetuating unhealthily weight gain, and being overweight making the degree of inflammation in the body worse.

Research has shown that turmeric and curcumin can interrupt this cycle by improving the inflammatory processes that are related to obesity. In addition, as you learned in the last chapter, research on diabetic patients' use of turmeric and curcumin has found that both substances can also help people who are overweight shed pounds, including excess abdominal weight, which is a serious risk factor for diabetes, cancer, heart disease, and other serious degenerative conditions. This is particularly true of curcumin.

Ongoing scientific research continues to demonstrate that curcumin helps promote weight loss and reduce the incidence of obesity-related diseases. Researchers have established that curcumin "directly interacts with white adipose tissue [body fat] to suppress chronic inflammation. In adipose tissue, curcumin inhibits macrophage infiltration and nuclear factor κB (NF-κB) activation induced by inflammatory agents." Curcumin has also been found to reduce the expression of potent pro-inflammatory cytokines, such as tumor necrosis factor-α (TNFα), that are also known to play a role in the onset of obesity.

Just as importantly, curcumin activates adiponectin, the primary anti-inflammatory compound secreted by adipocytes [fat cells that primarily make up adipose tissue]. Curcumin has also been shown to regulate lipid (fat) metabolism in the body, which, if disrupted, plays a central role in the development of obesity. Other research has established that curcumin improves insulin signaling and insulin resistance, and the body's utilization and disposal of glucose, further aiding in weight loss.

Curcumin has also been found to inhibit obesity even when fats in the diet are excessively consumed. In addition, curcumin can also inhibit fatty liver disease, a condition that is common in people who are overweight or obese. Moreover, curcumin's proven antioxidant properties also play important roles in aiding weight loss. "Through these diverse mechanisms," researchers note, "curcumin reduces obesity and curtails the adverse health effects of obesity."

Based on these findings, if you need to lose weight or simply want to avoid unhealthy weight gain, it makes good sense to consider adding a high quality curcumin supplement to your overall health regimen.

CONCLUSION

The health benefits turmeric and curcumin provide for helping to prevent and relieve many common and serious diseases are powerful testaments for why the regular use of turmeric to spice up your meals, along with taking a daily curcumin supplement, makes very good sense. Both measures are easy to implement and, as the scientific evidence shows, highly effective.

Now it's time for you to learn how to use turmeric and curcumin supplements, and what you need to look for when purchasing them. You will find those answers in the next chapter.

10

Using & Choosing Turmeric

In this chapter, you will learn how to most effectively make turmeric and curcumin part of your daily overall health routine. And you will also learn guidelines to follow when choosing turmeric and curcumin products. Let's start with turmeric first.

SELECTING AND USING TURMERIC

The first thing to consider when choosing a turmeric product is its quality. This is extremely important because many turmeric spice brands can contain pesticides, heavy metals, fillers, and other harmful additives, given that many of them originate outside of the United States, in countries such as China and India, where quality control measures are far less stringent that they are here. Always look for turmeric that is certified organic and check the packaging labels to make sure it contains only turmeric, and nothing else.

Cooking with Turmeric

Once you have selected a high quality turmeric spice, you can use it liberally on a variety of meals. It adds a wonderful flavor to rice and pasta, and can also be used in other dishes as well. It can be used in soups, omelet dishes, and as a flavoring for meat, lamb, and poultry. Turmeric also goes well with chickpea, lentil, and other legume dishes, and can even be used as a flavoring for salads.

To obtain the most benefit from turmeric, however, it is best to heat it up, rather than simply sprinkling it onto your food dishes, and to combine it with black pepper or ginger. That's because turmeric is poorly absorbed when consumed unheated and by itself. Heating it and combining it with black pepper or ginger, as is traditionally done in Ayurvedic cooking methods,

153

can significantly increase turmeric's bioavailability, meaning how well it is absorbed and utilized by the body.

Cooking turmeric with coconut oil or ghee, a type of butter, is also highly recommended, as this too will dramatically increase its bioavailability. In India, traditional curry dishes typically contain turmeric, black pepper or ginger, and coconut oil or ghee. These dishes are based on dietary recommendations prescribed by Ayurvedic medicine.

Making "Golden Milk"

Another tasty way to obtain the benefits of turmeric is to make a traditional Ayurvedic drink that is sometimes referred to as "golden milk." Ayurvedic practitioners consider golden milk to be a healing elixir. It is very easy to make. Simply add half a teaspoon each of organic turmeric powder and organic ginger powder to eight to twelve ounces of milk (if you are lactose intolerant, you can use almond or coconut milk) along with a pinch of nutmeg or cinnamon spice. Mix thoroughly, then heat the mixture in a pan for a few minutes, taking care not to let it boil. You want it to be warm to the taste, but not too hot. Once the mixture is warm, pour into a cup and drink it all before it cools.

For a thicker version, you can also add a teaspoon of coconut oil or ghee butter to the mixture before you heat it. As a variation on golden milk, you can combine turmeric and ginger powder with coconut oil, and heat the mixture up, and then add it to smoothies. Over time, you will most likely find that golden milk leaves you feeling energized. For many people, it may also improve digestion.

Dosage and Storage

Turmeric has been found to be a very safe spice to consume, even at high doses (8,000 to 10,000 mg per day), which is far more than you are likely to consume each day even with liberal use of the spice. In some cases, however, too much turmeric has been known to cause gastrointestinal upset, so heed the signals your body gives you. If you experience such upsets, stop using turmeric for a day or two, and then lower the amount you use according to what your body can tolerate. Between each use, store turmeric powder at room temperature.

SELECTING AND USING CURCUMIN SUPPLEMENTS

As with turmeric, when it comes to choosing a curcumin product you should always opt for one that is of high quality. Avoid products that contain fillers and other additives and, if possible, choose products that are certified organic.

Finding a high quality curcumin supplement can be difficult if you don't know what to look for. For one thing, many curcumin products contain curcumin that is claimed to be "standardized to 95 percent." That sounds well and good, yet the problem is that such a claim says nothing whatsoever about whether or not their version of curcumin is well-absorbed. In many cases, the manufacturers use low-grade generic versions of curcumin that are very poorly absorbed. Therefore, look for products that state on their labels the level of bioavailability their curcumin has.

Manufacturers of high quality curcumin products often have their products independently tested by outside labs to ensure their products' quality and purity. Such tests not only measure curcumin's level of bioavailability, they also screen for the presence of harmful mycotoxins (fungi), pesticides (including glyphosate), heavy metals, industrial solvents, and other additives. You want to avoid all curcumin products that contain any of the above classes of harmful ingredients. Manufacturers whose curcumin products are shown by independent lab testing to be free of these contaminants will usually include a Certificate of Analysis verifying these findings on their websites. You can also email or call these companies if you have any questions.

Knowing the bioavailability of curcumin products is also very important. Curcumin on its own is also poorly absorbed by the body, just as turmeric is. Curcumin products that also contain black pepper extract (piperene, often labeled as BioPerine) help improve curcumin's bioavailability. The herb boswellia serrata, also known as frankincense, can also significantly improve curcumin absorption, and is often an ingredient in high quality curcumin supplements.

Look to see whether either of these ingredients is included in the curcumin formulation you are considering.

Some manufacturers also make use of customized curcumin extracts that have been proven to have much higher bioavailability that other forms of curcumin. Such customized forms of curcumin include BCM-95, Longvida Optimized Curcumin Extract, and Meriva. All of these customized forms have been shown to increase curcumin bioavailability by as much as 1,000 percent or more.

Another highly absorbable type of curcumin supplement is one that is combined with liposomes. Liposomes are spherical substances composed of one or more layers of phospholipids (a class of fats) that have been shown to dramatically enhance the delivery to and absorption of nutrients and pharmaceutical drugs the body's cells. Liposomal curcumin products have been shown to be up to 185 times more absorbable than generic curcumin.

Finally, you may be interested in obtaining the same type of curcumin supplement that caused the woman with incurable stage four multiple myeloma that you read about in Chapter 4 to achieve and maintain a complete remission of her cancer for more than five years. The brand she used contained a proprietary curcumin formula known as Curcumin C3, so called because it contains curcumin, along with the curcuminoids demethoxycurcumin (DMC) and bisdemethoxycurcumin (BDMC) in a specific ratio. Curcumin C3 is manufactured and trademarked by Muhammed Majeed, PhD, founder of the Sabinsa Corporation, which licenses this product for use to a number of supplement companies here in the United States, as well as other nutritional companies around the world.

Dosage and Storage

Research has shown that high quality curcumin supplements can be effective at a daily dose of 400 mg. A typical dose range for such supplements is 400 to 1,000 mg of bioavailable curcumin. However, like turmeric itself, curcumin supplements are generally safe, even when taken in doses of up to 8,000 mg per day. For best results, start out with a lower dose and then scale up to a higher dose if need be, until you begin to notice consistent benefits. In cases of arthritis, brain conditions, chronic pain, cancer, and diabetes, a daily dose in the higher range limit may be necessary.

Curcumin supplements can be taken either with or away from meals. To further enhance their bioavailability, you can try taking them with organic coconut oil, measuring between a teaspoon to a tablespoon. For most people, the best time to take curcumin supplements is in the morning so that the benefits they provide are available throughout the rest of the day.

As with all other nutritional and herbal supplements, before taking curcumin supplements, please consult with your physician, especially if you are also using pharmaceutical drugs. If you are, you should also consider avoiding curcumin supplements that contain BioPerine or other black pepper extracts, because they not only enhance the bioavailability of curcumin, but can also increase the absorption of such medications, potentially causing unhealthy drug interactions. Curcumin can also interfere with the effectiveness of chemotherapy drugs, as well as anti-platelet drugs, and anticoagulants.

As with most other nutritional supplements, curcumin supplements can be stored at room temperature without any need for refrigeration. They should also be used before their expiration date, which will be listed on the bottle.

CONCLUSION

As this chapter makes clear, both turmeric and curcumin are extremely easy and safe to use. The key is to choose high quality forms of both substances. Look for curcumin products that are both pure and have high bioavailability. For turmeric, insist on using only brands that are certified organic, and use it in conjunction with other spices and oils that enhance its absorbability.

For best results, heat turmeric spice by adding it to the dishes and soups that you prepare. To get the greatest benefits, consider using turmeric in many of your daily meals while also taking a daily, high-quality curcumin supplement.

Conclusion

Now that you have read this far, you know of the many important health benefits that both turmeric and curcumin can provide for you and your loved ones. What you do with the knowledge you have gained from reading this book is, of course, up to you. My hope is that you will put it to good use by applying what you have learned.

The next step is up to you. I encourage you to experiment with adding turmeric as a spice in the meals you prepare, following the guidelines that you learned about in Chapter 10. Also see what happens when you add golden milk to your diet.

I also encourage you to start taking a high-quality curcumin supplement once a day. Doing so may be one of the most important self-care steps you can take to protect yourself from many of the most serious and difficult-to-treat diseases plaguing so many men, women, and children today.

Remember: The only way that you will know for sure if turmeric and curcumin can improve your health is to begin using them on a regular basis. If you are willing to do so, and also willing to follow an overall healthy diet and lifestyle, I think you will soon find that both substances will go a long way towards helping to ensure your good health. And in the case of turmeric, it will also add delicious flavoring to your meals.

Thank you very much for reading this book. I greatly appreciate your taking the time to do so.

Health and Blessings!

Resources

The following companies manufacture or supply high-quality brands of organic turmeric spice and bioavailable curcumin.

Organic Turmeric Spice
Aadi Organics, LLC
(832) 235-6103
www.aadiorganics.com
Supplier of organic spices, including turmeric, ginger, and chili powders.

Banyan Botanicals
(800) 953-6424
www.banyanbotanicals.com
Supplier of Ayurvedic herbs, oils, spices, and supplements.

Feel Good Organics, LLC
www.feelgoodorg.com
Supplier of organic herbs and spices.

Jiva Organics
(604) 254-9480
www.jivaorganics.ca
Supplier of organic, vegetarian, gluten-free health foods.

Mountain Rose Herbs
(800) 879-3337
www.mountainroseherbs.com
Supplier of organic herbs, spices, teas, and essential oils.

Naturevibe Botanicals
www.naturevibe-botanicals.com
Supplier of organic herbs and spices.

New Chapter
(888) 874-4461
www.newchapter.com
Supplier of multivitamins and supplements.

North American Herbs and Spice
(800) 243-5242
www.northamericanherbandspice
 .com
Supplier of herbs, spices, essential oils, and other supplements.

Opportuniteas
(513) 760-0035
www.opportuniteas.com
Supplier of organic and vegan supplements.

Organic Traditions
https://organicpowerfoods.com
Supplier of organic foods, drinks, and supplements.

Organic Wise
(877) 412-5961
www.organic-wise.com
Supplier of organic herbs and
supplements.

Sari Foods Company
(800) 590-8737
https://sarifoods.co/
Supplier of organic supplements.

Simply Organic c/o Frontier
Co-op
(800) 717-4372
www.simplyorganic.com
Supplier of organic spices and
seasonings.

Starwest Botanicals
(800) 800-4372
www.starwest-botanicals.com
Supplier of organic herbs, spices,
teas, and essential oils.

The Organique Co
(888) 988-5922
www.theorganiqueco.com
Supplier of organic superpowders.

Z!NT
(877) 290-4346
www.zintnutrition.com
Supplier of organic supplements.

ZNatural Foods
(888) 963-6637
www.znaturalfoods.com
Supplier of natural, organic foods
and supplements.

Curcumin Supplements
1MD
(888) 393-4030

https://1md.org
Supplier of health supplements.

BioOptimal
(800) 210-4863
www.biooptimalsupplements.com
Supplier of organic supplements.

Health Wise
(800) 395-8931
www.healthwisenri.com
Supplier of health-focused foods and
dietary supplements.

Life Extension
(800) 678-8989
www.lef.org
Supplier of vitamins and minerals,
supplements, and herbs.

Nature's Way
(800) 962-8873
www.naturesway.com
Supplier of vitamins and minerals,
herbs, and probiotics.

Nature Wise
(800) 510-7207
www.naturewise.com
Supplier of natural supplements.

North American Herbs and
Spice
(800) 243-5242
www.northamericanherbandspice
.com
Supplier of herbs, spices, essential oils,
and other supplements.

Planetary Herbals
(800) 606-6226
www.planetaryherbals.com
Supplier of natural dietary supplements.

Precision Naturals

www.precisionnaturals.com

Supplier of natural dietary supplements.

PuraTHRIVE

(888) 292-8309

http://purathrive.com

Supplier of vitamins and dietary supplements.

Sabinsa Corporation

(732) 777-1111

www.sabinsa.com

Supplier of dietary supplements and other nutritional products. Sabinsa manufactures the proprietary Curcumin C3 formulation that I wrote about in Chapter 10. You can find a listing of the nutritional supplement companies that are licensed by Sabinsa to use Curcumin C3 in their curcumin products at www.curcuminoids.com/index.php/curcuminc3users.

References

Chapter 1

Davidson, Alan. *The Oxford Companion to Food.* Oxford: Oxford UP, 1999. Print.

"First Curry Powder Advert." *First Curry Powder Advert.* British Library Board, n.d. Web. 09 Feb. 2015.

Prance, Ghillean T., and Mark Nesbitt. *The Cultural History of Plants.* New York.: Routledge, 2005. Print.

Ravindran, P. N., K. Nirmal Babu, and K. Sivaraman. *Turmeric: The Genus Curcuma.* Boca Raton, FL: CRC, 2007. Print.

Saberi, Helen, and Colleen Taylor Sen. *Turmeric: Great Recipes Featuring the Wonder Spice That Fights Inflammation and Protects Against Disease.* Chicago: Agate Digital, 2014.

Chapter 2

Ahmadi N, Eshaghian S, Huizenga R, et al. "Effects of intense exercise and moderate caloric restriction on cardiovascular risk factors and inflammation." *Am J Med.* 2011;124(10):978–82.

Arney K. "The LOX enzyme—Preparing the ground for cancer spread." *Cancer Research UK.* Jan 7, 2009. Available at http://scienceblog.cancerresearchuk.org/2009/01/07/the-lox-enzyme-preparing-the-ground-for-cancer-spread.

Arnson, Y., Shoenfeld, Y., and Amital, H. "Effects of tobacco smoke on immunity, inflammation and autoimmunity." *J. Autoimmun.* 2010;34(3):J258–65.

Bastard, J.-P., Maachi, M., Lagathu, C., et al. "Recent advances in the relationship between obesity, inflammation, and insulin resistance." *Eur. Cytokine Netw.* 2006;17(1):4–12.

Bonsall DR and Harrington ME (2013) "Circadian rhythm disruption in chronic fatigue syndrome." *Advances in Neuroimmune Biology,* 4 (2013) 265–274.

Centers for Disease Control and Prevention. FASTSTATS—Leading Causes of Death. cdc.gov. 2011; Available at: http://www.cdc.gov/NCHS/fastats/Default.htm.

Chainani-Wu, N. Safety and anti-inflammatory activity of curcumin: a component of turmeric (Curcuma longa). *J Altern Complement Med.* 2003;9(1):161–168.

Coccaro EF et al. "Elevated Plasma Inflammatory Markers in Individuals With Intermittent Explosive Disorder and Correlation With Aggression in Humans." *JAMA Psychiatry.* Feb. 2014;71(2):158–165.

Cretu E, Trifan A, Vasincu A, Miron A. "Plant-derived anticancer agents—curcumin in cancer prevention and treatment." *Rev Med Chir Soc Med Nat Iasi.* 2012 Oct-Dec;116(4):1223–9.

Deshpande, R., Khalili, H., Pergolizzi, R. G., Michael, S. D., and Chang, M. D. "Estradiol down-regulates LPS-induced cytokine production and NFkB activation in murine macrophages." *Am. J. Reprod. Immunol.* 1997;38(1):46–54.

Dixon WG, Bansback N. "Understanding the side effects of glucocorticoid therapy: shining a light on a drug everyone thinks they know." *Ann Rheum Dis .* 2012 Nov;71(11):1761–4.

Flynn DL, Rafferty MF, Boctor AM. "Inhibition of 5-hydroxy-eicosatetraenoic acid (5-HETE) formation in intact human neutrophils by naturally-occurring diarylheptanoids: inhibitory activities of curcuminoids and yakuchinones." *Prostaglandins Leukot Med.* 1986 Jun; 22(3):357–60.

Fried, S. K., Bunkin, D. A., and Greenberg, A. S. "Omental and subcutaneous adipose tissues of obese subjects release interleukin-6: depot difference and regulation by glucocorticoid." *J Clin Endocrinol Metab.* 1998;83(3):847–850.

Galland, L. Diet and inflammation. *Nutr Clin Pract.* 2010;25(6):634–640.

Gilliver, S. C. Sex steroids as inflammatory regulators. J. *Steroid Biochem. Mol. Biol.* 2010;120(2–3):105–115.

Harrington ME (2012) Neurobiological studies of fatigue. *Prog. Neurobiol.* 99: 93–105.

Keller, E. T., Chang, C., and Ershler, W. B. "Inhibition of NFkappaB activity through maintenance of IkappaBalpha levels contributes to dihydrotestosterone-mediated repression of the interleukin-6 promoter." *J Biol Chem.* 1996;271(42):26267–26275

Kundu, J. K., and Surh, Y.-J. "Inflammation: gearing the journey to cancer." *Mutat Res.* 2008;659(1–2):15–30.

Lee, J., Taneja, V., and Vassallo, R. "Cigarette Smoking and Inflammation: Cellular and Molecular Mechanisms." *J. Dent. Res.* 29 Aug 2011;91(2):142–149.

Menon VP, Sudheer AR. "Antioxidant and anti-inflammatory properties of curcumin." *Adv Exp Med Biol.* 2007;595:105–25.

Murphy SL. et al. Deaths: Preliminary Data for 2010. National Vital Statistics Report 60:4; 1/11/2012.

Ortega Martinez de Victoria, E., Xu, X., Koska, J., et al. "Macrophage content in subcutaneous adipose tissue: associations with adiposity, age, inflammatory markers, and whole-body insulin action in healthy Pima Indians." *Diabetes.* 2009; 58(2):385–393.

Pervanidou, P., and Chrousos, G. P. "Metabolic consequences of stress during childhood and adolescence." *Metab. Clin. Exp.* 2011;61:611–619.

Peterson K, McDonagh M, Thakurta S, et al. "Drug Class Review: Nonsteroidal Antiinflammatory Drugs (NSAIDs): Final Update 4 Report." National Institute of Health (NIH) PubMed Health. Bethesda (MD): National Library of Medicine (US). Nov 2010.

Ravindranath V, Chandrasekhara N. "*In vitro* studies on the intestinal absorption of curcumin in rats. "*Toxicology.* 1981;20:251–7.

Ray, P., Ghosh, S. K., Zhang, D. H., and Ray, A. "Repression of interleukin-6 gene expression by 17 beta-estradiol: inhibition of the DNA-binding activity of the transcription factors NF-IL6 and NF-kappa B by the estrogen receptor." *FEBS letters.* 1997;409(1):79–85.

Raison CL, Miller AH. "Is Depression an Inflammatory Disorder?" *Curr Psychiatry Rep.* 2011 Dec;13(6):467–475.

Sahebkar, A. (2014), "Are Curcuminoids Effective C-Reactive Protein-Lowering Agents in Clinical Practice? Evidence from a Meta-Analysis." *Phytother. Res.* 28: 633–642. doi:10.1002/ptr.5045

Schrager, M. A., Metter, E. J., Simonsick, E., et al. "Sarcopenic obesity and inflammation in the InCHIANTI study." *J Appl Physiol.* 2007;102(3):919–925.

Sharma RA, Euden SA, Platton SL, et al. "Phase I clinical trial of oral curcumin: Biomarkers of systemic activity and compliance." *Clin Cancer Res.* 2004;10:6847–54.

Singh, T., and Newman, A. B. "Inflammatory markers in population studies of aging." *Ageing Res Rev.* 2011;10(3):319–329.

Trayhurn, P., and Wood, I. S. "Signalling role of adipose tissue: adipokines and inflammation in obesity." *Biochem. Soc. Trans.* 2005;33(Pt 5):1078–1081.

Uribarri J, Cai W, Sandu O, Peppa M, Goldberg T, Vlassara H. "Diet-derived advanced glycation end products are major contributors to the body's AGE pool and induce inflammation in healthy subjects." *Ann N Y Acad Sci.* 2005 Jun;1043:461–6.

Vgontzas, A. N., Papanicolaou, D. A., Bixler, E. O., et al. "Sleep apnea and daytime sleepiness and fatigue: relation to visceral obesity, insulin resistance, and hypercytokinemia." *J Clin Endocrinol Metab.* 2000;85(3):1151–1158

Vgontzas, A. N., Papanicolaou, D. A., Bixler, E. O., Kales, A., Tyson, K., and Chrousos, G. P. "Elevation of plasma cytokines in disorders of excessive daytime sleepiness: role of sleep disturbance and obesity." *J Clin Endocrinol Metab.* 1997;82(5):1313–1316

Vgontzas, A. N., Zoumakis, M., Bixler, E. O., et al. "Impaired nighttime sleep in healthy old versus young adults is associated with elevated plasma interleukin-6 and cortisol levels: physiologic and therapeutic implications." *J Clin Endocrinol Metab.* 2003;88(5):2087–2095

Weisberg, S. P., McCann, D., Desai, M., Rosenbaum, M., Leibel, R. L., and Ferrante, A. W. "Obesity is associated with macrophage accumulation in adipose tissue." *J Clin Invest.* 2003;112(12):1796–1808.

White, B., and Judkins, D. Z. "Clinical Inquiry. Does turmeric relieve inflammatory conditions?" *J Fam Pract.* 2011;60(3):155–156

Windgassen, E. B., Funtowicz, L., Lunsford, T. N., Harris, L. A., and Mulvagh, S. L. "C-reactive protein and high-sensitivity C-reactive protein: an update for clinicians." *Postgrad Med.* 2011;123(1):114–119.

Woo, HM et al. "Active spice-derived components can inhibit inflammatory responses of adipose tissue in obesity by suppressing inflammatory actions of macrophages and release of monocyte chemoattractant protein-1 from adipocytes." *Life Sci.* 2007 Feb 13;80(10):926–31.

Yaffe, K., Lindquist, K., Penninx, B. W., et al. "Inflammatory markers and cognition in well-functioning African-American and white elders." *Neurology.* 2003;61(1):76–80.

Young, NA et al. "Oral administration of nano-emulsion curcumin in mice suppresses inflammatory-induced NFκB signaling and macrophage migration." *PloS One.* 2014 Nov 4;9(11):e111559.

Yuan, G., Wahlqvist, M. L., He, G., Yang, M., and Li, D. "Natural products and anti-inflammatory activity." *Asia Pac J Clin Nutr.* 2006;15(2):143–152.

Chapter 3

Bassin EB. (2001). "Association Between Fluoride in Drinking Water During Growth and Development and the Incidence of Ostosarcoma for Children and Adolescents." Doctoral Thesis, Harvard School of Dental Medicine. p. 15.

Begum AN *et al.* "Curcumin structure-function, bioavailability, and efficacy in models of neuroinflammation and Alzheimer's disease." *J Pharmacol Exp Ther.* 2008; 326:196–208.

Chhavi S et al. "Curcumin attenuates neurotoxicity induced by fluoride: An *in vivo* evidence." *Pharmacogn Mag.* 2014 Jan-Mar;10(37):61–65.

Cox KH et al. "Investigation of the effects of solid lipid curcumin on cognition and mood in a healthy older population." *J Psychopharmacol.* 2015 May;29(5):642–51.

Department of Health and Human Services. (1991). "Review of fluoride: benefits and risks. Report of the Ad Hoc Subcommittee on Fluoride." Washington, DC. p. 70.

Dong Z, et al. (1993). "Determination of the contents of amino-acid and monamine neurotransmitters in fetal brains from a fluorosis-endemic area." *Journal of Guiyang Medical College* 18(4):241–45.

Du L. (1992). "The effect of fluorine on the developing human brain." *Chinese Journal of Pathology* 21(4):218–20; republished in *Fluoride* 2008, 41(4):327–330.

Erciyas K, Sarikaya R. (2009). "Genotoxic evaluation of sodium fluoride in the Somatic Mutation and Recombination Test (SMART)." *Food & Chemical Toxicology* 47(11):2860–2.

Goozee KG, Sha TM, et al. "Examining the potential clinical value of curcumin in the prevention and diagnosis of Alzheimer's disease." *Brit J. Nutr* (2016), 115, 449–465.

He H, et al. (1989). "Effects of fluorine on the human fetus. *"Chinese Journal of Control of Endemic Diseases* 4(3):136–138, 1989; republished in *Fluoride* 2008, 41(4):321–326.

Hishikawa N, Takahashi Y et al. "Effects of turmeric on Alzheimer's disease with behavioral and psychological symptoms of dementia." *Ayu.* 2012 Oct-Dec; 33(4): 499–504.

Kunz D, et al. (1999). "A new concept for melatonin deficit: on pineal calcification and melatonin excretion." *Neuropsychopharmacology* 21(6):765–72.

Lim GP, Chu T, et al "The curry spice curcumin reduces oxidative damage and amyloid pathology in an Alzheimer transgenic mouse." *J. Neurosci.*, 2001, 21, 8370–8377.

Lopresti AL, Maes M, Maker GL, et al. "Curcumin for the treatment of major depression: A randomised, double-blind, placebo controlled study." *J Affect Dis.* 2014; 167:368–375.

Lopresti AL, Maes M, Meddens MJ, et al. "Curcumin and major depression: a randomised, double-blind, placebo-controlled trial investigating the potential of peripheral biomarkers to predict treatment response and antidepressant mechanisms of change." *Eur Neuropsychopharmacol.* 2015; 25(1):38–50.

Lu X, Deng Y et al. "Histone Acetyltransferase p300 Mediates Histone Acetylation of PS1 and BACE1 in a Cellular Model of Alzheimer's Disease." *PloS One.* 2014; 9(7): e103067.

Luke J. (2001). "Fluoride deposition in the aged human pineal gland." *Caries Res.* 35(2):125–128.

Luke J. (1997). "The Effect of Fluoride on the Physiology of the Pineal Gland." Ph.D. Thesis. University of Surrey, Guildford.

Ma QL et al. "Curcumin suppresses soluble tau dimers and corrects molecular chaperone, synaptic, and behavioral deficits in aged human tau transgenic mice." *J Biol Chem.* 2013; 288:4056–4065.

Mahlberg R, et al. (2009). "Degree of pineal calcification (DOC) is associated with polysomnographic sleep measures in primary insomnia patients." *Sleep Med.* 10(4):439–45.

Marier J, Rose D. (1977). "Environmental Fluoride. National Research Council of Canada. Associate Committee on Scientific Criteria for Environmental Quality." NRCC No. 16081.

Mihashi M, Tsutsui T. (1996). "Clastogenic activity of sodium fluoride to rat vertebral body-derived cells in culture." *Mutation Research.* 368(1):7–13.

National Toxicology Program [NTP] (1990). "Toxicology and Carcinogenesis Studies of Sodium Fluoride in F344/N Rats and B6C3fl Mice." *Technical Report Series No. 393.* NIH Publ. No 91-2848. National Institute of Environmental Health Sciences, Research Triangle Park, N.C.

Pandav R, Belle SH, DeKosky ST. "Apolipoprotein E polymorphism and Alzheimer's disease: The Indo-US cross-national dementia study." *Arch Neurol.* 2000;57:824–30.

Thiyagarajan M. and Sharma SS. "Neuroprotective effect of curcumin in middle cerebral artery occlusion induced focal cerebral ischemia in rats." *Life Sci.*, 2004, 74, 969–985.

Tiwari H, Rao MV. (2010). "Curcmin supplementation protects from genotoxic effects of arsenic and fluoride." *Food & Chemical Toxicology.* 48(5):1234–8.

Tooth Decay. Fluoride Action Network. http://fluoridealert.org/issues/caries/who-data

Vajragupta, O et al. "Manganese complexes of curcumin andits derivatives: evaluation for the radical scavenging ability and neuroprotective activity." *Free Radic. Biol. Med.*, 2003, 35, 1632–1644.

Yaffe, K., Lindquist, K., Penninx, B. W., et al. "Inflammatory markers and cognition in well-functioning African-American and white elders." *Neurology.* 2003;61(1):76–80.

BB, Kumar A, Bharti AC. "Anticancer potential of curcumin: preclinical and clinical trials." *Anticancer Res* Yu JJ, Pei LB, Zhang Y, et al. Chronic supplementation of curcumin enhances the efficacy of antidepressants in major depressive disorder: a randomized, double-blind, placebo-controlled pilot study. *J Clin Psychopharmacol.* 2015;35(4):406–410.

Yu Y, et al. (1996). "Neurotransmitter and receptor changes in the brains of fetuses from areas of endemic fluorosis." *Chinese Journal of Endemiology* 15:257–259; re-published in *Fluroide* 2008, 41(2):134–138.

Chapter 4

Abe Y, Hashimoto S, Horie T. "Curcumin inhibition of inflammatory cytokine production by peripheral blood monocytes and alveolar macrophages." *Pharmacol Res.* 1999;39:41–47.

Aggarwal. "Anticancer potential of curcumin: Preclinical and clinical studies." *Anticancer Res.* 2003;23(1A):363–398.

Aggarwal, BB, Shishodia S, Sandur SK, Pandey MK, and Sethi, G. "Inflammation and cancer: how hot is the link?" *Biochem. Pharmacol.* 2006;72(11):1605–1621.

Angelo LS, Kurzrock R. "Tumeric and green tea: a recipe for the treatment of B-chronic lymphocytic leukemia." *Cancer Res.* 2009;15(4):1123–1125.

Arbiser JL, Klauber N, Rohan R, et al. "Curcumin is an in vivo inhibitor of angiogenesis." *Mol Med.* 1998;4(6):376–383.

Bakshi J, Weinstein L, Poksay KS, et al. "Coupling endoplasmic recticulum stress to the cell death program in mouse melanoma cells: the effect of curcumin." *Apoptosis.* 2008;13(7):904–914.

Banerji A, Chakrabati J, Mitra A, Chatterjee A. "Effect of curcumin on gelatinase A (MMP-2) activity in B16F10 melanoma cells." *Cancer Lett.* 2004;211(2):235–242.

Betancor-Fernandez A, Perez-Galvez A, Sies H, et al. "Screening pharmaceutical preparations containing extracts of turmeric rhizome, artichoke leaf, devil's claw root, garlic or salmon oil for antioxidant capacity." *J Pharm Pharmacol.* 2003;55(3):981–986.

Bhandarkar SS, Arbiser JL. "Curcumin as an inhibitor of angiogenesis." *Adv Exp Medi Biol.* 2007;595:185–195.

Bill MA, Bakan C, Benson DM, et al. "Curcumin induces proapoptotic effects against human melanoma cells and modulates the cellular response to immunotherapeutic cytokines." *Mol Cancer Ther.* 2009;8(9):2726–2735.

Bonte F. et al. "Protective effect of curcuminoids on epidermal skin cells under free oxygen radical stress." *Planta Medica.* 1997;63:265–66.

Cancer Facts and Figures 2017. American Cancer Society. www.cancer.org/research/cancer-facts-statistics/all-cancer-facts-figures/cancer-facts-figures-2017.html

Cancer Statistics. National Cancer Institute. www.cancer.gov/about-cancer/understanding/statistics

Chadalapaka G, Jutoor I, Chitharlapalli S, et al. "Curcumin decreases specificity protein expression ib bladder cancer cells." *Cancer Res.* 2008;68(13):5345–5354.

Cheah YH, Nordin FJ, Sarip R, et al. "Combined xanthorrhizol-curcumin exhibits synergistic growth inhibitory activity via apoptosis induction in human breast cancer cells MDA-MD-231." *Cancer Cell Int.* 2009;2:1.

Chen Y, Wu Y, He J, Chen W. "The experimental and clinical study on the effect of curcumin on cell cycle proteins and regulating proteins of apoptosis in acute myelogenous leukemia." *J Huazhong Univ Sci Technol Med Sci.* 2002;22:295–298.

Chuang SE. Kuo ML, Hsu CH, et al. "Curcumin-containing diet inhibits diethylnitrosamine-induced murine hepatocarcinogenesis." *Carcinogenesis.* 2000; 21:331–335.

Chuang SE, Cheng AL, Lin JK, et al. "Inhibition by curcumin of diethylnitrosamine-induced hepatic hyperplasia, inflammation, cellular gene products and cell-cycle-related proteins in rats." *Food Chem Toxicol.* 2000;38:991–995.

Ciolino HP, Daschner PJ, Wang TT, Yeh GC. "Effect of curcumin on the aryl hydrocarbon receptor and cytochrome P450 1A1 in MCF-1 human breast carcinoma cells." *Biochem Pharmacol.* 1998;56(2):197–206.

Deeb DD, Jiang H, Gao X, et al. "Chemosensitization of hormone-refractory prostate cancer cells by curcumin to TRAIL-induced apoptosis." *J Exp Ther Oncol.* 2005;5(2):81–91.

Deshpande SS, Maru GB. "Effects of curcumin on the formation of benzo-pyrene derived DNA adducts in vitro." *Cancer Letters.* 1995;96:71–80.

Dickinson DA, Levonen AL, Moellering DR, et al. "Human glutamate cysteine ligase gene regulation through the electrophile response element." *Free Radic Biol Med.* 2044;37(8):1152–1159.

Dickinson DA, Iles KE, Zhang H, et al. "Curcumin alters EpRE and AP-1 binding complexes and elevates glutamate-cysteine ligase gene expression." *Faseb J.* 2003;17(3):473–475.

Sharma RA, Gescher AJ, Steward WP. "Curcumin: The story so far." *Eur J Cancer.* 2005;41(13)1955–1968.

Duvoix A, Blasius R, Delhalle S, et al. "Chemopreventive and therapeutic effects of curcumin." *Cancer Lett.* 2005;223(2):139–145.

Duvoix A, Morceau F, Schnekenburger M, et al. "Curcumin-induced cell death in two leukemia cell lines: K562 and Jurkat." *Ann NY Acad Sci.* 2003;1010:389–392.

Fuller B, Dijk S, Butler P, et al. "Pro-inflammatory agents accumulate during donor liver cold preservation: A study on increased adhesion molecule expression and abrogation by curcumin in cultured endothelial cells." *Cryobiology.* 2003;46:284–288.

Garcea G, Berry DP, Jones DJ, et al. "Consumption of the putative chemopreventive agent curcumin by cancer patients: assessment of curcumin levels in the colorectum and their pharmacodynamic consequences." *Cancer Epidemiol Biomarkers Prev.* 2005;14(1):120–125.

Gescher A, Pastorino U, Plummer SM, Manson TM. "Suppression of tumor development by substances derived from the diet-mechanisms and clinical implications." *Br J Clin Pharmacol.* 1998;45(1):1–12.

Gupta B, Ghosh B. "Curcuma longa inhibits TNF-alpha-induced expression of adhesion molecules on human umbilical vein endothelial cells." *Int J Immunopharmacol.* 1999;21:745–757.

Friedman L, Lin L, Ball S, et al. "Curcumin analogues exhibit enhanced growth suppressive activity in human pancreatic cancer cells." *Anticancer Drugs.* 2009;20(6):444–449.

Hammamieh R, Sumaida D, Zhang X, et al. "Control of the growth of human breast cancer cells in culture by manipulation of arachidonate metabolism." *BMC Cancer.* 2007;7:138.

Hauser PJ, Han Z, Sindhwani P, et al. "Sensitivity of bladder cancer cells to curcumin and its derivatives depends on the extracellular matrix." *Anticancer Res.* 2007;27(2):737–740.

Hong J, Bose M, Ju J, et al. "Modulation of arachidonic acid metabolism by curcumin and related beta-diketone derivatives: effects on cytosolic phospholipase A(2),cyclooxygenases and 5-lypoxygenase." *Carcinogenesis.* 2004;25:1671–1679.

Huang TY, Tsai TH, Hsu CW, et al. "Curcuminoids suppress the growth and induce apoptosis through caspase-3-dependent pathways in glioblastoma multiforme (GBM) 8401 cells." *J. Agric. Food Chem.* 2010;58(19):10639–10645.

Iqbal M, Sharma SD, Okazaki Y, et al. "Dietary supplementation of curcumin enhances antioxidant and phase II metabolizing enzymes in ddY male mice: possible role in protection against chemical carcinogenesis and toxicity." *Pharmacol Toxicol.* 2003;92(1):33–38.

Inano H, Onoda N, Inafuku M, et al. "Potent preventive action of curcumin on radiation-induced initiation of mammary tumorigenesis in rats." *Carcinogenesis.* 2000; 21:1835–1841.

Johnson JJ, Mukhtar H. "Curcumin for chemoprevention of colon cancer." *Cancer Lett.* 2007;255(2):170–181.

Johnson SM, Gulhati P, Arrieta I, et al. "Curcumin inhibits proliferation of colorectal carcinoma by modulating Akt/mTOR signaling." *Anticancer Res.* 2009;29(8): 3185–3190.

Kunnumakkara AB, Anand P, Aggarwal BB. "Curcmin inhibits proliferation, invasion, angiogenesis and metastasis of different cancer through interaction with multiple signaling proteins." *Cancer Lett.* 2008;269(2):199–225.

Kuo ML, Huang TS, Lin JK. "Curcumin, an antioxidant and anti-tumor promoter, induces apoptosis in human leukemia cells." *Biochem Biophys Acta.* 1996;1317:95–100.

Lalitha S, Selvam R. "Prevention of H2Os-induced red blood cell lipid peroxidation by aqueous extracted turmeric." *Asia Pacific J Clin Nutr.* 1999;8(2):113–14.

Lee J, Im YH, Jung HH, et al. "Curcumin inhibits interferon-alpha-induced NF-kappaB and COX-2 in human A549 non-small cell lung cancer cells." *Biochem Biophys Res Commun.* 2005;334:313–318.

Lin JK, Shih CA. "Inhibitory effect of curcumin on xanthine dehydrogenase/oxidase induced by phorbol-12-myristate-13-acetate in NIH3T3 cells." *Carcinogenesis.* 1994;15:1717–2171.

Liontas A, Yeger H. "Curcumin and resveratrol induce apoptosis and nuclear translocation and activation of p53 in human neuroblastoma." *Anticancer Res.* 2004;24:987–988.

LoTempio MM, Veena MS, Steele HL, et al., "Curcumin suppresses growth of head and neck squamous cell carcinoma." *Clin Cancer Res.* 2005;11(19 Pt 1):6994–7002.

Maheshwari RK, Singh AK, Gaddipati J, et al. "Multiple biological activities of curcumin: a short review." *Life Sci.* 2006;78(18):2081–2087.

Milacic V, Banerjee S, Landis-Piwowar KR, et al. "Curcumin inhibits the proteasome activity in human colon cancer cells in vitro and in vivo." *Cancer Res.* 2008;68(18):7283–7292.

Miller M, Chen S, Woodruff J, et al. "Curcumim (diferuloymethane) inhibits cell proliferation, induces apoptosis, and decreases hormone levels and secretion in pituitary cancer cells." *Endocrinology.* 2008;149(8):4158–4167.

Nagai S, Kurimoto M, Washiyama K, et al., "Inhibition of cellular proliferation and induction of apoptosis by curcumin in human malignant astrocytoma cell lines." *J Neurooncol.* 2005;74(2):105–11.

Nakamura Y, Ohto Y, Murakami A, et al. "Inhibitory effects of curcumin and tetrahydrocurcuminoids on the tumor promoter-induced reactive oxygen species in leukocytes in vitro and invivo." *Jpn J Cancer Res.* 1998;89:-361–370.

Okada K, Wangpoentrakul C, Tanaka T, et al. "Curcumin and especially tetrahydrocurcumin ameliorateoxidative stress-induced renal injury in mice." *J Nutr.* 2001;131:2090–2095.

Phan TT, See P, Lee ST, et al. "Protective effects of curcumin against oxidative damage on skin cells in vitro: its implication for wound healing." *J Trauma.* 2001;51:927–931.

Reddy AC, Lokesh BR. "Effect of dietary turmeric (*Curcuma longa*) on iron-induced lipid preoxidation in the rat liver." *Food Chem Toxicol.* 1994;32:279–283.

Rogers, Lois. "How curry spice helped a dying woman beat cancer: Sufferer, 67, turned to kitchen cupboard staple turmeric after five years of failed treatment." *Daily Mail* 25 July 2017.

Rowe DL, Ozbay T, O'Regan RM, Nahta R. "Modulation of the BRCA1 protein and induction of apoptosis in triple negative breast cancer cell lines by the polyphenolic compound curcumin." *Breast Cancer.* 2009;3:61–75.

Sahu Rp, Batra S, Srivastava SK. "Activation of ATM/Chk1 by curcumin causes cell cycle arrest and apoptosis in human pancreatic cancer cells." *Br J Cancer.* 2009;100(9):1425–1433.

Selvam R, Subramanian L, Gayathri R, Angayarkanni N. "The anti-oxidant activity of turmeric (*Curcuma longa*)." *J Ethnopharmacol.* 1995;47:59–67.

Shankar S, Chen Q, Sarva K, et al. "Curcumin enhances the apoptosis-inducing potential of TRAIL in prostate cancer cells: molecular mechanisms of apoptosis, migration and angiogenesis." *J Mol Signal.* 2007;2:10.

Shankar S, Ganapathy S, Chen Q, et al. "Curcumin sensitizes TRAIL-resistant xenografts: molecular mechanisms of apoptosis, metastasis and angiogenesis." *Mol Cancer.* 2008;7:16.

Teiten MH, Gaascht F, Eifes S, et al. "Chemopreventive potential of curcumin in prostate cancer." *Genes Nutr.* 2010;5(1):64–74.

Sharma OP. "Antioxidant activity of curcumin and related compounds." *Biochem Pharmacol.* 1976;25:1811–1812.

Shukla Y, Arora A. "Suppression of altered hepatic foci development by curcumin in wistar rats." *Nutr Cancer.* 2003;45:53–59.

Singh S. Aggarwal BB. "Activation of transcription factor NF-kappa B is suppressed by curcumin (diferuloylmethane) [corrected]." *J Biol Chem.* 1995;270:24,995–25,000.

Singh SV, Hu X, Srivastava SK, et al. "Mechanism of inhibition of ebnzo[A] pyrene-induced forestomach cancer in mice by dietary curcumin." *Carcinogenesis.* 1998;19(8):1357–1360.

Soudamini KK, Unnikrishnan MC, Soni, KB. Kuttan R. "Inhibition of lipid per-oxidation and cholesterol levels in mice by curcumin." *Indian J Physiol Pharmacol.* 1992;36:239–243.

Sreejavan N, Rao MN. "Free radical scavenging activity of curcuminoids."*Arzneimit-telforschung.* 1996;46(2):169–171.

Sreejayan N, Rao MN. "Nitric oxide scavenging by curcuminoids." *J Pharm Pharmacol.* 1997;49(1):105–107.

Statistics For Different Kinds of Cancer. Centers for Disease Control and Prevention. www.cdc.gov/cancer/dcpc/data/types.htm.

Subramanian M., et al. "Diminution of singlet oxygen-induced DNA damage by curcumin and related antioxidants." *Mutation Research*. 1994;311:249–55.

Sudarshana P, Berliner A, Suraj SF, et al. "Curcumin blocks brain tumor formation." *Brain Research*. 2009;1266:130–138.

Sun C, Liu X, Chen Y, et al., "Anticancer effect of curcumin on human B cell non-Hodgkin's lymphoma." *J Huazhong Univ Sci Technolog Med Sci*. 2005;25(4):404–7.

Sung B, Kunnumakkara AB, Sethi G, Anand P, et al. "Curcumin circumvents chemoresistance in vitro and potentiates the effect of thalidomide and bortezomib against human multiple myeloma in nude mice model." *Mol Cancer Ther*. 2009;8(4):959–970.

Surh YJ, Chun KS. "Cancer chemopreventive effects of curcumin." *Adv Exp Med Biol*. 2007;595:149–172.

Thaloor D, Singh AK, Sidhu GS, et al. "Inhibition of angiogenic differentiation of human umbilical vein endothelial cells by curcumin." *Cell Grwoth Differ*. 1998;9(4):305–312.

Thapliyal R, Maru GB. "Inhibition of cytochrome P450 isozymes by curcumin in vitro and in vivo." *Food Cehm Toxicol*. 2001;39(6):541–547.

Tomita M, Holman BJ, Santoro CP et al. "Astrocyte production of the chemokine macrophage inflammatory protein-2 is inhibited by the spice principle curcumin at the level of gene transcription." *J Neuroinflammation*. 2005;2:8.

Van Erk MJ, Teuling E, Staal YC, et al. "Time- and dose-dependent effects of curcumin on gene expression in human colon cancer cells." *J Carcinog*. 2004;3(1):8.

Verma SP, Salamone E, Goldin BR. "Curcumin and genistein, plant natural products, show synergistic inhibitory effects on the growth of human breast cancer MCF-7 cells induced by estrogenic pesticides." *Biochem Biophys Res Commun*. 1997;233(3):692–696.

Verma SP, Goldin BR, Peck SL. "The Inhibition of Estrogenic Effects of Pesticides and Environmental Chemicals by Curcumin and Isoflavonoids." *Environ Health Perspectives*. 1998;106(12):807–812.

Wang X, Wang Q, Ives, Kl, Evers BM. "Curcumin inhibits neurotensin-mediated interleukin-8 production and migration of HCT116 human colon cancer cells." *Clin Cancer Res*. 2006;12(18):5346–5355.

Wang Z, Desmoulin S, Banerjee S, et al. "Synergistic effects of multiple natural products in pancreatic cancer cells." *Life Sci*. 2008;83(7–8):293–300.

Wu Y, Chen Y, Chen W. "Effects of concurrent use of rh-IFN-gamma and curcumin on the anti-proliferative capacity of HL-60 cells." *J Tongji Med Univ*. 1999;19:267–270.

Wu LX, Xu JH, Wu, CH, Chen YZ. "Inhibitory effect of curcumin on proliferation of

K562 cells involves down-regulation of p210(bcr/abl) initiated Ras signal transduction pathway." *Acta Pharmacol Sin.* 2003;24:1155–1160.

Yu Y, Kanwar SS, Patel BB, et al. "Elimination of colon cancer stem-like cells by the combination of curcumin and FOLFOX." *Transl Oncol.* 2009;2(4):321–328.

Zaidi A, Lai M, Cavanagh J. "Long-term stabilisation of myeloma with curcumin." *BMJ Case Reports.* 16 April 2017, doi:10.1136/bcr-2016–218148.

Zhang HG, Kim H, Liu C, et al. "Curcumin reverses breast tumor exosomes mediated immune suppression of NK cell tumor cytotoxicity." *Biochem Biophys Acta.* 2007;1773(7):1116–1123.

Chapter 5

American Heart Association's *Heart Disease and Stroke Statistics—2012 Update.Coronary Heart Disease: The Dietary Sense and Nonsense* edited by Dr. George V. Mann, M.D., New York:Veritas Society, 1993.

Akazawa N et al. "Curcumin ingestion and exercise training improve vascular endothelial function in postmenopausal women." *Nutrition Research*—17 October 2012. Published online ahead of print. doi: 10.1016/j.nutres.2012.09.002.

Akazawa N et al. "Effects of curcumin intake and aerobic exercise training on arterial compliance in postmenopausal women." *Artery Research.* 28 September 2012 (10.1016/j.artres.2012.09.003)

Basta G, Schmidt AM, De Caterina R. "Advanced glycation end products and vascular inflammation: implications for accelerated atherosclerosis in diabetes." *Cardiovasc Res.* 2004 Sep 1;63(4):582–92.

Cho JW, Lee KS, Kim GW. "Curcumin attenuate the expression of IL-1β, IL-6, and TNF-α as well as cyclin E in TNF-α-treated HaCaT cell; NF-kB and MAPKs as potential upstream targets." *Int J Mol Med.* 2007;19:469–474.

Gavin KM, Seals DR, Silver AE, Moreau KL. "Vascular endothelial estrogen receptor alpha is modulated by estrogen status and related to endothelial function and endothelial nitric oxide synthase in healthy women." *J Clin Endocrinol Metab.* 2009;94:3513–3520.

Herrera MD, Mingorance C, Rodríguez-Rodríguez R, Alvarez de Sotomayor M. "Endothelial dysfunction and aging: an update. Ageing Res Rev. 2010;9:142–152 La Vecchia C. Sex hormones and cardiovascular risk." *Hum Reprod.* 1992;7:162–167.

Petrusson H et al. "Is the use of cholesterol in mortality risk algorithms in clinical guidelines valid? Ten years prospective data from the Norwegian HUNT 2 study." *J of the Eval of Clin Pract.* 2012:18(1):159–168.

Qin S, Huang L, et al. "Efficacy and safety of turmeric and curcumin in lowering blood lipid levels in patients with cardiovascular risk factors: a meta-analysis of randomized controlled trials." *Nutr J* 2017 Oct 11;16(1):68.

Quiles JL, Mesa MD, Ramírez-Tortosa CL, Aguilera CM, Battiono M, Gil A, et al.

"Curcuma longa extract supplementation reduces oxidative stress and attenuates aortic fatty streak development in rabbits." *Arterioscler Thromb Vasc Biol.* 2002;22:1225–1231.

Ramsen CE et al. "Re-evaluation of the traditional diet-heart hypothesis: analysis of recovered data from Minnesota Coronary Experiment (1968–73)." *BMJ* 12 April 2016;353:i1246.

Ravnskov U, et al. "Lack of an association or an inverse association between low-density-lipoprotein cholesterol and mortality in the elderly: a systematic review." *BMJ Open* 2016;6:e010401.doi:10.1136/bmjopen-2015–010401.

Sugawara J, Akazawa N, Miyaki A, Choi Y, Tanabe Y, Imai T, Maeda S. "Effect of endurance exercise training and curcumin intake on central arterial hemodynamics in postmenopausal women: pilot study." *Am J Hypertens.* 2012 Jun;25(6):651–6. doi: 10.1038/ajh.2012.24. Epub 2012 Mar 15.

Sumbilla, C., Lewis, D., Hammerschmidt, T. and Inesi, G., "The slippage of the Ca2+ pump and its control by anions and curcumin in skeletal and cardiac sarcoplasmic reticulum." *Biol. Chem.*, 2002, 277, 13900–13906.

Taddei S, Virdis A, Ghiadoni L, Mattei P, Sudano I, Bernini G, et al. "Menopause is associated with endothelial dysfunction in women." *Hypertension.* 1996;28:576–582.

Thijssen DH, Black MA, Pyke KE, Padilla J, Atkinson G, Harris RA, et al. "Assessment of flow-mediated dilation in humans: a methodological and physiological guideline." *Am J Physiol Heart Circ Physiol.* 2011;300:H2–H12.

Wongcharoen W, Phrommintikul A. "The protective role of curcumin in cardiovascular diseases." *Int J Cardiol.* 2009 Apr 3;133(2):145–51.

Chapter 6

Abreu, MT, Fukata M, and Breglio K. "Innate Immunity and its Implications on Pathogenesis of Inflammatory Bowel Disease." [ed.] Stephan R. Targan, Fergus Shanahan and Loren C. Karp. *Inflammatory Bowel Disease: Translating Basic Science Into Clinical Practice.* West Sussex: John Wiley and Sons: Blackwell Publishing Ltd, 2010, 7, pp. 64–81.

Aljamal A. "Effects of Turmeric in Peptic Ulcer and Helicobacter pylori." *Plant Sciences Research.* 2011;3:25–28.

Amani S et al. "Natural products in treatment of ulcerative colitis and peptic ulcer." *Journal of Saudi Chemical Society.* January 2013;17:101–124.

Aggarwal, Bharat B., et al., et al. "Curcumin—Biological and Medicinal Properties." [ed.] P. N. Ravindran, K. Nirmal Babu and K. Sivaraman. *Turmeric: The Genus Curcuma.* Boca Raton: CRC Press: Taylor & Francis Group, 2007, 10, pp. 298–348.

Aggarwal BB. "Do dietary spices impair the patient-reported outcomes for stapled hemorrhoidopexy? A randomized controlled study." *Surgical Endoscopy,* May 2011;25:1535–1540.

Altomare DF et al. "Red Hot Chili Pepper and Hemorrhoids: The Explosion of a Myth: Results of a Prospective, Randomized, Placebo-Controlled, Crossover Trial." *Diseases of the Colon & Rectum*. July 1, 2006;49(7):1018–1023.

Baljinder S et al. "Antimicrobial Potential of Polyherbo-Mineral Formulation Jatyadi Taila—A Review." *International Journal of Research in Ayurveda and Pharmacy*. Jan-Feb 2011;2:151–156.

Balakrishnan, K.V. "Postharvest Technology and Processing of Turmeric." *Turmeric: The Genus Curcuma*. Boca Raton: CRC Press: Taylor & Francis Group, LLC, 2007, 8, pp. 193–256.

Bernstein, Charles N. "Epidemiology of Inflammatory Bowel Disease: the Shifting Landscape." [ed.] Stephan R. Targan, Fergus Shanahan and Loren C. Karp. *Inflammatory Bowel Disease: Translating Basic Science Into Clinical Practice*. West Sussex: John Wiley and Sons: Blackwell Publishing Ltd, 2010, 3, pp. 9–15.

Bharat B et al. "Molecular Targets of Nutraceuticals Derived from Dietary Spices: Potential Role in Suppression of Inflammation and Tumorigenesis." *Experimental Biology and Medicine*. 1 Aug 2009;234(8):825–849.

Binion, David G. and Rafiee, Parvaneh. "Inflammatory Bowel Disease Microcirculation and Diversion, Diverticular and Other Non-infectious Colitides. [ed.] Stephan R. Targan, Fergus Shanahan and Loren C. Karp." *Inflammatory Bowel Disease: Translating Basic Science Into Clinical Practice*. West Sussex: John Wiley and Sons: Blackwell Publishing Ltd, 2010, 42, pp. 609–618.

Bundy R *et al.* "Turmeric Extract May Improve Irritable Bowel Syndrome Symptomology in Otherwise Healthy Adults: A Pilot Study." *The Journal Of Alternative And Complementary Medicine*. 2004;10(6):1015–1018.

Carabotti M et al. "The gut-brain axis: interactions between enteric microbiota, central and enteric nervous systems." *Ann Gastroenterol*. 2015 Apr-Jun; 28(2): 203–209.

Chattopadhyay I et al. "Turmeric and curcumin: Biological actions and medicinal applications." *Curr Sci*. 10 Jul 2004;87:44–53.

Coon, JT and Ernst, E. "Herbal medicinal products for non-ulcer dyspepsia." *Alimentary Pharmacology & Therapeutics*. 19 Sept. 2002;16:1689–1699.

Duke, James A., Bogenschutz-Godwin, Mary Jo and duCellier, Judi. *CRC Handbook of Medicinal Spices*. Boca Raton: CRC Press LLC, 2003.

Elson, Charles O. and Weaver, Casey T. "In Vivo Models of Inflammatory Bowel Disease. [ed.] Stephan R. Targan, Fergus Shanahan and Loren C. Karp." *Inflammatory Bowel Disease: Translating Basic Science Into Clinical Practice*. West Sussex: John Wiley and Sons: Blackwell Publishing Ltd, 2010, 5, pp. 25–51.

Epstein, J., Docena, G., Macdonald, T. T., and Sanderson, I. R. "Curcumin suppresses p38 mitogen-activated protein kinase activation, reduces IL-1beta and matrix metalloproteinase-3 and enhances IL-10 in the mucosa of children and adults with inflammatory bowel disease." Br J Nutr. 2010;103(6):824–832.

Goldman, Alan L. *The Evaluation of Rectal Pain and Bleeding and The Non-Operative*

Treatment of Hemorrhoids and Anal Fissures. Atlanta: Emory University: The Center for Colorectal Health, 2007.

Gupta, Meva Lal, Gupta, S.K. and Bhuyan, Chaturbhuja. [ed.] "Comparative clinical evaluation of Kshara Sutra ligation and hemorrhoidectomy in Arsha (hemorrhoids)." *International Quarterly Journal of Research in Ayurveda.* Apr-Jun 2011;32:225–229.

Kim D-C et al. "Curcuma longa Extract Protects against Gastric Ulcers by Blocking H2 Histamine Receptors." *Biol & Pharmaceut Bulletin.* December 2005;28:2220–4.

Koosirirat C et al. "Investigation of the anti-inflammatory effect of Curcuma longa in Helicobacter pylori-infected patients." *Int Immunopharmacol.* July 2010;10:815–818.

Krzyzanowska J et al. "Dietary Phytochemicals and Human Health." *Bio-Farms for Nutraceuticals: Functional Food and Safety Control by Biosensors.* Austin: Landes Bioscience and Springer Science+Business Media, LLC, 2010, 7, pp. 74–98.

Lang A et al. "Curcumin in Combination With Mesalamine Induces Remission in Patients With Mild-to-Moderate Ulcerative Colitis in a Randomized Controlled Trial." *Clin Gastroenterol Hepatol* 2015 Aug;13(8):1444–9.

Langmead, Louise and Rampton, David S. "Complementary Medicine. [ed.] Stephan R. Targan, Fergus Shanahan and Loren C. Karp." *Inflammatory Bowel Disease: Translating Basic Science Into Clinical Practice.* West Sussex: John Wiley and Sons: Blackwell Publishing Ltd, 2010, 48, pp. 693–704.

Mayo Clinic staff. Inflammatory bowel disease (IBD): Risk factors; Treatments and drugs. *Mayo Foundation for Medical Education and Research.* February 18, 2015.

Murray, Michael T. and Pizzorno, Joseph E. "Curcuma longa (turmeric)." *Textbook of Natural Medicine.* 2. Edinburgh: Harcourt Publishers Limited: Churchill Livingstone, 1999, pp. 690–694.

Nahar, Lutfun and Sarker, Satyajit D. "Phytochemistry of the Genus Curcuma. [ed.] P. N. Ravindran, K. Nirmal Babu and K. Sivaraman." *Turmeric: The Genus Curcuma.* Boca Raton: CRC Press: Taylor & Francis Group, LLC, 2007, 3, pp. 71–106.

Pattiyathanee P, Vilaichone R, "Chaichanawongsaroj N. Effect of curcumin on Helicobacter pylori biofilm formation." *African Journal of Biotechnology.* 9 Oct 2009;8(19):5106–5115.

Prucksunand C et al. Phase II "Clinical Trial on Effect of the Long Turmeric (Curcuma Longa Linn) on Healing of Peptic Ulcer." *The Southeast Asian Journal of Tropical Medicine and Public Health.* Mar 2001;32:208–215.

Rajasekaran SA. "Therapeutic potential of curcumin in gastrointestinal diseases." *World J Gastroenterol.* 15 Feb 2011;2:1–14.

Reddy Y. et al. "Studies on Chemistry and Biological Activities of Curcuma Longa Linn—A Review." *Int J Advances Pharmaceut Res.* 24 Jan 2011;2:26–36.

Remadevi, R., Surendran, E. and Kimura, Takeatsu. "Turmeric in Traditional Medicine." [ed.] *Turmeric: The Genus Curcuma.* Boca Raton: CRC Press: Taylor & Francis Group, 2007, 12, pp. 409–436.

Rogler, Gerhard. "Non-targeted Therapeutics for Inflammatory Bowel Diseases." *Inflammatory Bowel Disease: Translating Basic Science Into Clinical Practice.* West Sussex: John Wiley and Sons: Blackwell Publishing Ltd, 2010, 24.

Sarker, Satyajit D. and Nahar, Lutfun. "Bioactivity of Turmeric." [ed.] *Turmeric: The Genus Curcuma.* Boca Raton: CRC Press: Taylor & Francis Group, LLC, 2007, 9, pp. 258–285.

Song WB et al. "Curcumin Protects Intestinal Mucosal Barrier Function of Rat Enteritis via Activation of MKP-1 and Attenuation of p38 and NF-αB Activation." *PLoS One.* 2010 Sep 24;5(9):e12969.

Sushil K et al. [ed.] "Curcumin for maintenance of remission in ulcerative colitis." Cochrane IBD Group. s.l.: John Wiley & Sons, Ltd., October 17, 2012, Cochrane Database of Systematic Reviews.

Swarnakar S et al., "Curcumin Regulates Expression and Activity of Matrix Metalloproteinases 9 and 2 during Prevention and Healing of Indomethacin-induced Gastric Ulcer." *J Biol Chem.* 11Mar 2005:280:9409–9415.

Taylor RA, Leonard MC "Curcumin for Inflammatory Bowel Disease: A Review of Human Studies." *Alternative Medicine Review.* June 2011;16:152–156.

The Brain-Gut Connection. www.hopkinsmedicine.org/health/healthy_aging/healthy_body/the-brain-gut-connection#.

Van Dau N et al. "The effects of a traditional drug, turmeric (Curcuma longa), and placebo on the healing of duodenal ulcer." *Phytomedicine.* March 1998;5:29–34.

Yoon S et al. "Management of Irritable Bowel Syndrome (IBS) in Adults: Conventional and Complementary/Alternative Approaches." *Alternative Medicine Review* June 2011;16:134–51.

Chapter 7

Ahn K. Kim S et al. "Metabolomic Elucidation of the Effects of Curcumin on Fibroblast-Like Synoviocytes in Rheumatoid Arthritis." *PloS One.* 2015 Dec 30;10(12):e0145539.

Amalraj A, Varma K et al. "A Novel Highly Bioavailable Curcumin Formulation Improves Symptoms and Diagnostic Indicators in Rheumatoid Arthritis Patients: A Randomized, Double-Blind, Placebo-Controlled, Two-Dose, Three-Arm, and Parallel-Group Study." *J Med Food.* 2017 Oct;20(10):1022–1030.

Chainani-Wu, N. "Safety and anti-inflammatory activity of curcumin: a component of turmeric (Curcuma longa)." *J Altern Complement Med.* 2003;9(1):161–168.

Chandran B, Goel A: "A randomized, pilot study to assess the efficacy and safety of curcumin in patients with active rheumatoid arthritis." *Phytother Res* 2012;26:1719–1725.

Daily JW, Yang M, Park S. "Efficacy of Turmeric Extracts and Curcumin for Alleviating the Symptoms of Joint Arthritis: A Systematic Review and Meta-Analysis of Randomized Clinical Trials." *J Med Food.* 2016 Aug 1; 19(8): 717–729.

DiPiero F et al. "Comparative evaluation of the pain-relieving properties of a lecithinized formulation of curcumin (Meriva(®)), nimesulide, and acetaminophen." *J Pain Res*.2013;6:201–5.

Fu M, Chen L, Zhang L, Yu X, Yang Q. "Cyclocurcumin, a curcumin derivative, exhibits immune-modulating ability and is a potential compound for the treatment of rheumatoid arthritis as predicted by the MM-PBSA method." *Int J Mol Med*. 2017 May;39(5):1164–1172.

Funk JL, Frye JB, Oyarzo JN, et al. : "Efficacy and mechanism of action of turmeric supplements in the treatment of experimental arthritis." *Arthritis Rheum* 2006;54:3452–3464.

He Y, Yue Y, Zheng X, Zhang K, Chen S, Du Z: "Curcumin, inflammation, and chronic diseases: How are they linked?" *Molecules* 2015;20:9183–9213.

Kuptniratsaikul V, Dajpratham P, Taechaarpornkul W, et al. : "Efficacy and safety of *Curcuma domestica* extracts compared with ibuprofen in patients with knee osteoarthritis: A multicenter study." *Clin Interv Aging* 2014;9:451–458.

Kuptniratsaikul V, Thanakhumtorn S, Chinswangwatanakul P, Wattanamongkonsil L, Thamlikitkul V: "Efficacy and safety of *Curcuma domestica* extracts in patients with knee osteoarthritis." *J Altern Complement Med* 2009;15:891–897.

Madhu K, Chanda K, Saji MJ: "Safety and efficacy of *Curcuma longa* extract in the treatment of painful knee osteoarthritis: A randomized placebo-controlled trial." *Inflammopharmacology* 2013;21:129–136.

Menon V.P., Sudheer A.R. "Antioxidant and anti-inflammatory properties of curcumin." *Adv. Exp. Med. Biol.* 2007;595:105–125.

Mukherjee D, Nissen SE, Topol EJ: "Risk of cardiovascular events associated with selective COX-2 inhibitors." *JAMA* 2001;286:954–959.

Nakagawa Y, Mukai S, Yamada S, et al. : "Short-term effects of highly-bioavailable curcumin for treating knee osteoarthritis: A randomized, double-blind, placebo-controlled prospective study." *J Orthop Sci* 2014;19:933–939.

Panahi Y, Rahimnia AR, Sharafi M, Alishiri G, Saburi A, Sahebkar A: "Curcuminoid treatment for knee osteoarthritis: A randomized double-blind placebo-controlled trial." *Phytother Res* 2014;28:1625–1631.

Panahi Y., Alishiri G.H., Parvin S., Sahebkar A. "Mitigation of systemic oxidative stress by curcuminoids in osteoarthritis: Results of a randomized controlled trial." *J. Diet. Suppl.* 2016;13:209–220.

Peddada KV, Peddada KV, Shukla SK, Mishra A, Verma V: "Role of curcumin in common musculoskeletal disorders: A review of current laboratory, translational, and clinical data." *Orthop Surg* 2015;7:222–231.

Pinsornsak P, Niempoog S: "The efficacy of *Curcuma longa* L. extract as an adjuvant therapy in primary knee osteoarthritis: A randomized control trial." *J Med Assoc Thai* 2012;95 Suppl 1:S51–S58.

Priyadarsini K.I., Maity D.K., Naik G.H., Kumar M.S., Unnikrishnan M.K., Satav J.G., Mohan H. "Role of phenolic O-H and methylene hydrogen on the free radical reactions and antioxidant activity of curcumin." *Free Radic. Biol. Med.* 2003;35:475–484.

Ramadan G, Al-Kahtani MA, El-Sayed WM. "Anti-inflmmatory and anti-oxidant properties of Curcuma longa (turmeric) versus Zingiber officinale (ginger) rhizomes in rat adjuvant-induced arthritis." *Inflammation.* 2011 Aug;34(4):291–301.

Sahebkar A., Serbanc M.C., Ursoniuc S., Banach M. "Effect of curcuminoids on oxidative stress: A systematic review and meta-analysis of randomized controlled trials." *J. Funct. Foods.* 2015;18:898–909.

Suokas AK, Sagar DR, Mapp PI, Chapman V, Walsh DA: "Design, study quality and evidence of analgesic efficacy in studies of drugs in models of OA pain: A systematic review and a meta-analysis." *Osteoarthritis Cartilage* 2014;22:1207–1223.

White, B., and Judkins, D. Z. "Clinical Inquiry. Does turmeric relieve inflammatory conditions?" *J Fam Pract.* 2011;60(3):155–156.

Chapter 8

Abdel Aziz MT et al. "The effect of a novel curcumin derivative on pancreatic islet regeneration in experimental type-1 diabetes in rats (long term study)" *Diabetol Metab Syndr.* Nov 26, 2013;5:75.

Appendino G et al. "Potential role of curcumin phytosome (Meriva) in controlling the evolution of diabetic microangiopathy. A pilot study." *Panminerva Med.* 2011 Sep;53(3 Suppl 1):43–9.

Banafshe HR et al. "Effect of curcumin on diabetic peripheral neuropathic pain: possible involvement of opioid system." *Eur J Pharmacol.* Effect of curcumin on diabetic peripheral neuropathic pain: possible involvement of opioid system. 2014 Jan 15;723:202–6.

CDC: National Diabetes Statistic Report, 2017. Available at www.CDC.gov.

Chuengsamarn S et al. "Curcumin Extract for Prevention of Type 2 Diabetes." *Diabetes Care* 2012 Nov; 35(11): 2121–2127.

Ghorbani Z et al. "Anti-hyperglycemic and insulin sensitizer effects of turmeric and its principle constituent curcumin." *Int J Endocrinol Metab.* 2014 Oct 1;12(4):e18081.

Hie M et al. "Curcumin suppresses increased bone resorption by inhibiting osteoclastogenesis in rats with streptozotocin-induced diabetes." *Eur J Pharmacol.* 2009 Oct 25;621(1–3):1–9.

Jin QH et al. "Curcumin improves expression of SCF/c-kit through attenuating oxidative stress and NF-κB activation in gastric tissues of diabetic gastroparesis rats." *Diabetol Metab Syndr.* 2013 Mar 1;5(1):12.

Kant V et al. "Antioxidant and anti-inflammatory potential of curcumin accelerated the cutaneous wound healing in streptozotocin-induced diabetic rats." *Int Immunopharmacol.* 2014 Jun;20(2):322–30.

Kantikar M et al. "Novel role of curcumin in the prevention of cytokine-induced islet death in vitro and diabetogenesis in vivo." *Br J Pharmacol.* 2008 Nov;155(5):702–13.

Li Y et al. "Curcumin attenuates diabetic neuropathic pain by downregulating TNF-α in a rat model." *Int J Med Sci.* 2013;10(4):377–81.

Naijil G et al. "Curcumin pretreatment mediates antidiabetogenesis via functional regulation of adrenergic receptor subtypes in the pancreas of multiple low-dose streptozotocin-induced diabetic rats." *Nutr Res.* 2015 Sep;35(9):823–33.

Nal X et al. "Curcuminoids exert glucose-lowering effect in type 2 diabetes by decreasing serum free fatty acids: a double-blind, placebo-controlled trial." *Molecular Nutrition & Food Research* 2012 August 29.

Nal X et al. "Curcuminoids Target Decreasing Serum Adipocyte-fatty Acid Binding Protein Levels in Their Glucose-lowering Effect in Patients with Type 2 Diabetes." *Biomed Environ Sci.* 2014 Nov;27(11):902–6.

Pan Y et al. "Inhibition of high glucose-induced inflammatory response and macrophage infiltration by a novel curcumin derivative prevents renal injury in diabetic rats." *Br J Pharmacol.* 2012 Jun;166(3):1169–82.

Rahimi HR et al. "The effect of nano-curcumin on HbA1c, fasting blood glucose, and lipid profile in diabetic subjects: a randomized clinical trial." *Avicenna J Phytomed.* 2016 Sep-Oct;6(5):567–577.

Steigerwalt R. Meriva®, "a lecithinized curcumin delivery system, in diabetic microangiopathy and retinopathy." *Panminerva Med.* 2012 Dec;54(1 Suppl 4):11–6.

Usharani P et al. "Effect of NCB-02, atorvastatin and placebo on endothelial function, oxidative stress and inflammatory markers in patients with type 2 diabetes mellitus: a randomized, parallel-group, placebo-controlled, 8-week study." *Drugs R.D.* 2008;9(4):243–50.

Yang H et al. "Curcumin attenuates urinary excretion of albumin in type II diabetic patients with enhancing nuclear factor erythroid-derived 2-like 2 (Nrf2) system and repressing inflammatory signaling efficacies." *Exp Clin Endocrinol Diabetes.* 2015 Jun;123(6):360–7.

Yang YS et al. "Lipid-lowering effects of curcumin in patients with metabolic syndrome: a randomized, double-blind, placebo-controlled trial." *Phytother Res.* 2014 Dec;28(12):1770–7.

Zhang D et al. "Curcumin and Diabetes: A Systematic Review." *Evid Based Complement Alternat Med.* 2013; 2013: 636053.

Chapter 9

Agarwal R, Goel SK, Behari JR. "Detoxification and antioxidant effects of curcumin in rats experimentally exposed to mercury." *J Applied Toxicol.* Mar 12, 2010;30: 457–468.

Ahmad B, Lapidus L. "Curcumin prevents aggregation in α-synuclein by increasing reconfiguration rate." *J Biol Chem.* 2012 Mar 16;287(12):9193–9.

Alappat L, Awad AB. "Curcumin and obesity: evidence and mechanisms." *Nutr Rev.* 2010 Dec;68(12):729–38.

Araujo CAC and Leon LL. "Biological activities of *Curcuma longa* L." *Mem. Inst. Oswaldo Cruz,* 2001: 96: 723–728.

BanerjeeA. and Nigam SS. "Antimicrobial efficacy of the essential oil *of Curcuma longa. Indian J. Med. Res.,"* 1978;68:864–866.

Biswas J et al. "Curcumin protects DNA damage in a chronically arsenic-exposed population of West Bengal." *Hum Exp Toxicol.* 2010 Jun;29(6):513–24.

Bradford PG. "Curcumin and obesity." *Biofactors.* 2013 Jan-Feb;39(1):78–87.

Bright JJ. "Curcumin and autoimmune disease." *Adv Exp Med Biol.* 2007;595:425–51.

Chattopadhyay I et al. "Turmeric and curcumin: Biological actions and medicinal applications" *Current Science.* July 10, 2004;87:44–53.

Chen D-Y et al. "Curcumin inhibits influenza virus infection and haemagluttination activity." *Food Chemistry.* 15 April 2010;119(4):1346–51.

Dairam A, Fogel R, Daya S, Limson JL. "Antioxidant and iron-binding properties of curcumin, capsaicin, and S-allylcysteine reduce oxidative stress in rat brain homogenate." *J Agric Food Chem.* 2008 May 14;56(9):3350–6.

Garcia-Nino WR and Pedraza-Chaverri J. "Protective effect of curcumin against heavy metals-induced liver damage." *Food Chem Toxicol.* July 2014;69:182–201.

Gokul G, Geeta Rv. "Effect of curcuma longa extract on biofilm formation by streptococcus mutans." *Asian J Pharmaceut Clin Res.* July 2017;10(7):186–7.

Hemmer B et al. "Multiple sclerosis-a coordinated immune attack across the blood brain barrier." *Curr Neurovasc Res.* 2004 Apr;1(2):141–50.

Heng MC, Song MK, Harker J, Heng MK. "Drug-induced suppression of phosphorylase kinase activity correlates with resolution of psoriasis as assessed by clinical, histological and immunohistochemical parameters." *Br J Dermatol.* 2000;143:937–949.

Huang YD et al. "Study on the preparation of zedoary turmeric oil spray and its anti-virus effects." *Zhong Yao Cai.* 2007 Mar;30(3):342–5.

Jagatha B et al. "Curcumin treatment alleviates the effects of glutathione depletion in vitro and in vivo: therapeutic implications for Parkinson's disease explained via in silico studies." *Free Radic Biol Med.* 2008 Mar 1;44(5):907–17.

Jiao Y et al. S. V. *Iron chelation in the biological activity of curcumin.* Free Radic.Biol. Med. 4–1-2006;40(7):1152–1160.

Jiao Y et al. *Curcumin, a cancer chemopreventive and chemotherapeutic agent, is a biologically active iron chelator.* Blood 1–8-2009;113(2):462–469.

Kim K et al. "Curcumin inhibits hepatitis C replication via suppressing the Akt-SREBP-1 pathway." *FEBS Lett.* 2010 Feb 19;584(4):707–12.

Kurd SK et al. "Oral curcumin in the treatment of moderate to severe psoriasis vulgaris: a prospective clinical trial." *J Am Acad Dermatol.* 2008;58:625–631.

Lapidus L. and Cameron L. "Curcumin shows promise in attacking Parkinson's disease." *Michigan State University Today,* Mar 20, 2012. Available at: http://msutoday.msu.edu/news/2012/curcumin-shows-promise-in-attacking-parkinson/

Mythri RB and Barath MM. "Curcumin: a potential neuroprotective agent in Parkinson's disease." *Curr Pharm Des.* 2012;18(1):91–9.

Pescosolido N et al. "Curcumin: therapeutic potential in ophthalmology." *Planta Med.* 2014 Mar;80(4):249–54.

Qureshi M et al. "Therapeutic potential of curcumin for multiple sclerosis." *Neurol Sci.* 2017 Oct 27. doi: 10.1007/s10072–017–3149–5.

Reddy AC and Lokesh BR. *Effect of dietary turmeric (Curcuma longa) on iron-induced lipid peroxidation in the rat liver.* Food Chem.Toxicol 1994;32(3):279–283.

Reddy AC and Lokesh BR. *Studies on the inhibitory effects of curcumin and eugenol on the formation of reactive oxygen species and the oxidation of ferrous iron.* Mol.Cell Biochem. 8–17–1994;137(1):1–8.

Shankar TN and Murthy VS, Effect of turmeric (*Curcuma longa*) fractions on the growth of some intestinal and pathogenic bacteria *in vitro. Indian J. Exp. Biol.,* 1979;17(12):1363–1366.

Sreejayan and Rao MNA. "Curcumin inhibits iron-dependent lipid peroxidation." *Int J Pharmaceut* 1993;100:93–97.

Srichairatanakool S et al. *Curcumin contributes to in vitro removal of non-transferrin bound iron by deferiprone and desferrioxamine in thalassemic plasma.* Med.Chem. 2007;3(5):469–474.

Sun J, Han J, Zhao Y, Zhu Q, Hu J. "Curcumin induces apoptosis in tumor necrosis factor-alpha-treated HaCaT cells." *Int Immunopharmacol.* 2012;13:170–174.

Thephinlap C, Phisalaphong C, Fucharoen S, Porter JB, Srichairatanakool S. "Efficacy of curcuminoids in alleviation of iron overload and lipid peroxidation in thalassemic mice." *Med Chem.* 2009 Sep;5(5):474–82.

Thephinlap C, Phisalaphong C, Lailerd N, et al. "Reversal of cardiac iron loading and dysfunction in thalassemic mice by curcuminoids." *Med Chem.* 2011 Jan;7(1):62–9.

Tonnesen HH, de Vries H, Karlsen J, Beijersbergen van Henegouwen G. "Studies on curcumin and curcuminoids. IX: investigation of the photobiological activity of curcumin using bacterial indicator systems." *J Pharm Sci.* 1987;76:371–373.

Tuntipopipat S, Zeder C, Siriprapa P, and Charoenkiatkul S. *Inhibitory effects of spices and herbs on iron availability.* Int.J Food Sci.Nutr. 2009;60 Suppl 1:43–55.

Wang LL et al. "Curcumin, a potential therapeutic candidate for retinal diseases." *Mol Nutr Food Res.* 2013 Sep;57(9):1557–68.

Weijuan S et al. "Curcumin Prevents High Fat Diet Induced Insulin Resistance and Obesity via Attenuating Lipogenesis in Liver and Inflammatory Pathway in Adipocytes." *PLoS One.* 2012; 7(1): e28784.

Xie L, Li XK, Takahara S. "Curcumin has bright prospects for the treatment of multiple sclerosis." *Int Immunopharmacol.* 2011 Mar;11(3):323–30.

Xiu-fen L et al. "Curcumin, a potential candidate for anterior segment eye diseases: a review." *Front Pharmacol.* 2017 Feb 14;8:66.

Yu S et al. "Curcumin prevents dopaminergic neuronal death through inhibition of the c-Jun N-terminal kinase pathway." *Rejuvenation Res.* 2010 Feb;13(1):55–64.

Zbarsky V et al. "Neuroprotective properties of the natural phenolic antioxidants curcumin and naringenin but not quercetin and fisetin in a 6-OHDA model of Parkinson's disease." *Free Radic Res.* 2005 Oct;39(10):1119–25.

Acknowledgments

As always, my deepest thanks to, and appreciation for, my mother, brothers and sisters, and in particular, since being an uncle is one of my favorite roles in life, to my nieces and nephews and their children. And to my father, for the many important lessons he taught me by his example and for the way his spirit continues to guide me since his passing from this life, as well as to his older brother, my Uncle Nick, who in the past few years has also become a good friend of mine.

Once again, I am also deeply indebted to and grateful for all of my friends, without whom my life would be far less fun and love-filled. I want to especially thank those friends who have been there with and for me the longest, sharing their love, support, advice, and sense of humor in countless ways that have enriched my life. So a big shout out and my heartfelt thanks in equal measure to Ted Allen, Bob Cohen, Marc Smith, Richard Stark, and Paul Witte for everything that our friendship means to me.

This is the final book of what I jokingly refer to as my "food trilogy," which began with *Apple Cider Vinegar,* continued with *Coconuts For Your Health,* and now ends here. Like those other two books, this one would not have been written but for the suggestion of my friend and publisher, Rudy Shur. Thanks, Rudy. Thanks too, to your staff at Square One who were so helpful in shepherding this book all the way to its publication, especially my editor, Erica Shur.

Finally, a big hug and many thanks to Vladlena P., who from halfway around the world sparked my heart with the beauty of her smile.

About the Author

Larry Trivieri, Jr is a bestselling author and nationally recognized lay authority on holistic, integrative, and non-drug-based healing methods, with more than thirty years of personal experience in exploring techniques for optimal wellness and human transformation. During that time, Trivieri has interviewed and studied with over 400 of the world's top physicians and other health practitioners in over fifty disciplines in the holistic health field.

Trivieri is the author or co-author of over twenty-five books on health, including *Apple Cider Vinegar: Nature's Most Versatile and Powerful Remedy, Coconuts For Your Health, The Acid-Alkaline Lifestyle, The Acid-Alkaline Food Guide, Juice Alive, The American Holistic Medical Association Guide to Holistic Health, The Self-Care Guide to Holistic Medicine,* and *Outstanding Health: A Longevity Guide for Staying Young, Healthy, and Sexy for the Rest of Your Life.* He also served as editor and principal writer of both editions of the landmark health encyclopedia, *Alternative Medicine: The Definitive Guide,* and has written over 200 articles for Internet-based health sites. He has written numerous feature articles for a variety of publications, including *Alternative Medicine,* for which he served as contributing editor from 1999 through 2002; *Natural Health, Natural Solutions,* and *Yoga Journal.*

Trivieri is dedicated to sharing the wealth of potentially life-saving information he has learned about with as wide an audience as possible in order to help usher in a new era of wellness and health care in the twenty-first century. To that end, he also lectures about health nationwide, and has been a featured guest on numerous TV and radio shows across the United States.

Trivieri is also an acclaimed novelist and the author of *The Monster and Freddie Fype,* as well as the forthcoming titles *Krystle's Quest* and *Tommy's Big Question.* He lives in upstate New York.

You can learn more about and purchase his other books on Amazon.com using this link: http://amzn.to/2tDGSvu. You can also email him at larry-triv@write.me.

Index

Other Square One Titles of Interest

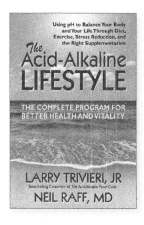

The Acid-Alkaline Lifestyle

The Complete Program for Better Health and Vitality

Larry Trivieri, Jr. and Neil Raff, MD

Why are so many of us afflicted with degenerative diseases? And why are the diseases that once plagued only the elderly, such as heart disease and diabetes, now increasingly affecting our younger generations? *The Acid-Alkaline Lifestyle* first provides a simple answer to these very important questions and then presents the first and only complete acid-alkaline balancing program—one that goes far beyond diet and nutrition. Here is the practical information you need to restore and maintain your health and boost your energy so that you can achieve a longer, healthier life, the way nature intended.

$17.95 US • 272 pages • 6 x 9-inch paperback • ISBN 978-0-7570-0389-9

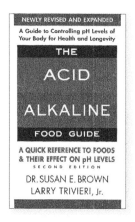

The Acid-Alkaline Food Guide

SECOND EDITION

A Quick Reference to Foods & Their Effect on pH Levels

Susan E. Brown, PhD, and Larry Trivieri, Jr.

Researchers around the world continue to report the importance of acid-alkaline balance. This book, now in its second edition, was designed as an easy-to-follow guide to the most common foods that influence your body's pH level. Updated information explores (and refutes) the myths about pH balance and diet, and guides you to supplements that can help you achieve a healthy pH level.

$8.95 US • 224 pages • 4 x 7-inch paperback • ISBN 978-0-7570-0393-6

Apple Cider Vinegar

Nature's Most Versatile and Powerful Remedy

Larry Trivieri, Jr.

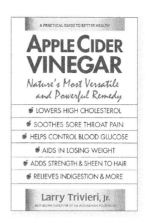

For centuries, apple cider vinegar has been used as a folk remedy to treat a host of health issues, from indigestion and low energy to sore throats and toothaches. As a beauty aid, it can help remove blemishes and add strength and sheen to hair. And that's just the tip of what this amazing elixir can do. Best-selling health author Larry Trivieri, Jr. has written this complete A-to-Z guide that shows how to use apple cider vinegar to prevent or reverse over eighty common health conditions, and to improve and maintain the health and appearance of your hair, skin, teeth, and gums.

$14.95 US • 240 pages • 6 x 9-inch paperback • ISBN 978-0-7570-0446-9

Coconuts for Your Health

Nature's Most Delicious & Effective Remedy

Larry Trivieri, Jr.

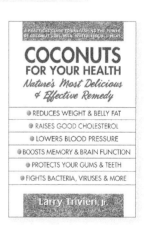

Before their introduction to the Standard Western Diet, natives of the South Pacific islands were among the healthiest people in the world. Heart disease and obesity were extremely rare, as were infectious diseases, dementia, and dental issues. Remarkably, the majority of calories consumed by these islanders came from coconuts. Today, medical researchers have rediscovered the many health benefits of this tropical fruit. Coconut has been found to raise good cholesterol, reduce belly fat, boost memory, protect teeth and gums, lower blood pressure, and more. This book focuses on specific concerns from heart disease to high blood pressure to memory loss, and explains how coconut works to combat these issues.

$15.95 US • 192 pages • 6 x 9-inch paperback • ISBN 978-0-7570-0451-3

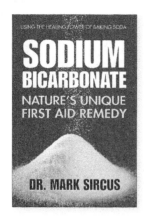

Sodium Bicarbonate

Nature's Unique First Aid Remedy

Dr. Mark Sircus

What if there were a natural health-promoting substance that was inexpensive and available at any grocery store? There is. It's called sodium bicarbonate, also known as baking soda. *Sodium Bicarbonate* begins with an overview of baking soda, chronicling its use as a home remedy. Author Mark Sircus then details how this extraordinary substance can alleviate a number of health disorders and suggests the most effective way to use sodium bicarbonate in the treatment of each condition. Let *Sodium Bicarbonate* help you look at baking soda in a whole new way.

$16.95 US • 208 pages • 6 x 9-inch paperback • ISBN 978-0-7570-0394-3

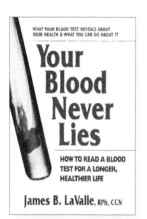

Your Blood Never Lies

How to Read a Blood Test for a Longer, Healthier Life

James B. LaValle, RPh, CCN

If you're like most people, you probably rely on your doctor to interpret the results of your blood tests, which contain a wealth of information on the state of your health. A blood test can tell you how well your kidneys and liver are functioning, your potential for heart disease and diabetes, the strength of your immune system, the chemical profile of your blood, and many other important facts about the state of your health. And yet, most of us cannot decipher these results ourselves, nor can we even formulate the right questions to ask about them—or we couldn't, until now. *Your Blood Never Lies* provides the up-to-date information you need to understand your results and take control of your life.

$16.95 US • 368 pages • 6 x 9-inch paperback • ISBN 978-0-7570-0350-9

For more information about our books,
visit our website at www.squareonepublishers.com